SILVER LEARNINGS

Practical Wisdom for Living with Brain Injury

CAROLE J. STARR, M.S.

Spiral Path Publishing
Scarborough, Maine

Spiral Path Publishing
spiralpathpublishing.com

Silver Learnings / Carole J. Starr
Print ISBN: 978-0-9986521-2-2
eBook ISBN: 978-0-9986521-3-9
Library of Congress Control Number: 2025914908

Book Cover Design by EbookLaunch.com

Disclaimer: This book references the author's personal experience living with brain injury. The author is not a medical or mental health professional. This book is not a substitute for health advice from a qualified professional. Readers should consult their own practitioners.

DEDICATION

I dedicate this book to everyone who has given me strength, hope, and encouragement through twenty-five years of living with brain injury.

Your impact lives within every word, every lesson, and every page of *Silver Learnings*.

Although the world is full of suffering,
it is also full of the overcoming of it.
—Helen Keller

TABLE OF CONTENTS

PREFACE

A Defining Milestone

Some events draw a hard line through our lives, marking a clear before and an after. They redefine who we are. Milestones like births, graduations, and marriages bring joy and promise. Others, like breakups, health crises, and deaths bring grief and devastation.

July 6th, 1999 is the defining milestone of my life. The day I sustained a brain injury in a car accident. The day when the life I knew and the life I expected, ended.

I was 32 years old. Like many people, I had identities I cherished. One of my most valued identities was *brain*. I was proud of my intellect, quick wit, and drive to achieve. I had been valedictorian of my high school class, graduated third in college, earned a master's degree in Adult Education and built a career as a self-employed corporate trainer. I worked hard but rarely struggled. I was a Type A, high achiever who was accustomed to excelling.

Teaching and music were two activities that had defined me since childhood. I tutored classmates beginning in third grade and started taking violin lessons in fourth. Nearly every job I'd held included an education role. I loved learning new material and figuring out creative ways to teach it.

Outside of work, I played violin in a community orchestra and sang soprano in a chorus. Music fed my soul in a way that nothing else did. While others cranked up rock, I turned up loud classical music. I planned to be an amateur musician forever.

Despite the joys these activities brought, there were aspects of my life I wanted to change. My hard-charging nature often led to perfectionism and overwork. While I loved teaching itself, I wasn't always passionate about the subjects I taught. I yearned for a life of purpose.

Also, as much as I loved music, time spent in orchestra and choral rehearsals and performances left little room for other social activities. Sometimes it felt like my life was on a treadmill going faster and faster, but not taking me anywhere. In hindsight, some kind of crash was inevitable. I just wish it hadn't been so literal.

On the day of the accident, I was driving from one teaching job to another when I was broadsided on the driver's side by a car going about 50 mph. The last thing I remember is the earsplitting sound of metal on metal. The airbags deployed, the windows shattered, and my car spun 180 degrees across the road. I don't remember any of those things, because I likely lost consciousness upon impact. I only know what happened because of the accident photos.

When I opened my eyes after the accident, the other driver was already at my window, yelling, *Get out! Get out! Get out!* I didn't understand why, but I obeyed. The driver's side door was crushed, so I had to crawl out through the passenger side. I stood in the middle of the road—dazed, confused, and unsteady. The sunlight seemed unnaturally bright. An off-duty paramedic stopped and helped me to the median to lie down and wait for the ambulance.

I was transported to the emergency room, a ride I don't remember. When asked if I'd hit my head, I said no, although my head did hurt. The doctor also asked if I remembered the accident. I confidently answered yes, unaware of how many details I was missing. I reported that I hadn't lost consciousness, which couldn't have been true. In my recollection, the other driver instantly appeared outside my window, yelling at me. In reality, I was probably unconscious during the time it took him to exit his vehicle and get to mine. I was diagnosed with severe whiplash and told I'd be fine in a few weeks.

It was the physical therapist treating my neck who first suspected a brain injury. My doctor confirmed I'd had a mild traumatic brain injury and said I should recover fully. I didn't know what mild traumatic brain injury meant and didn't think about it much at first. The screaming pain in my neck took priority. I assumed the brain issue would resolve on its own.

About six weeks later, the whiplash and other physical injuries had healed enough to attempt a slow return to my regular life. That's when everything fell apart.

The brain injury symptoms that had been mostly hidden by all the rest and support I'd been receiving suddenly exploded into my daily life. I was exhausted all the time. My head hurt constantly. It felt like someone was squeezing the left side of my brain from the inside. Sometimes it felt like the pressure would blow the top of my head off.

Teaching, where I had always felt competent and in control, became challenging, exhausting, and overstimulating. I forgot my students' names, even after multiple classes. I couldn't recall what topics we'd covered. The lesson plans I had written and used for years suddenly seemed too complicated to follow. Conversations moved too fast for me to keep up. I would leave students in groups long after they'd finished working because I was so overwhelmed. After just two hours of teaching, I would crash and spend two full days on the couch, too wiped out to do anything. I could barely handle just four hours of work a week.

Even simple tasks exhausted me. I had to nap every day after my morning shower because it drained me so much. I was too tired to even use the hair dryer, so I'd collapse on the couch with wet hair. This led to many memorable hair days.

I hoped returning to music and being bathed in sound would clear the mental fog that had invaded my brain. Instead, the previously comforting, familiar sounds of rehearsal had changed into a piercing cacophony that overloaded my brain. The normal pre-rehearsal mix of conversations and instruments was oddly and painfully loud.

When I opened my violin case and saw a broken string, I couldn't remember how to change it. I didn't even know where to sit, despite having had the same seat in that orchestra for ten years. I gritted my way through for five minutes, before the sound reduced me to tears and I ran from the room. I couldn't drive home, so a friend had to take me. It took days to recover from just a few minutes of music. It felt like the ultimate cruel joke to curse a musician with an intolerance to sound.

Eventually, I learned my extreme sound sensitivity had a name—hyperacusis. The effects impacted my whole life. Everyday noises felt magnified. Planes flying overhead made me duck, even when I was inside. Alarms made me scream and sometimes fall.

I also struggled with basic life tasks. In the grocery store, I would stand frozen in the produce section, unable to decide between two apples. One day I spent 30 minutes staring at shelves of bread, panicking because my usual brand was out of stock. I called my mother, crying, because I couldn't figure out what to buy. Food spoiled in the fridge because following a recipe and pulling together a meal was impossible. I ate cottage cheese for dinner most nights because I couldn't figure out what else to eat.

Reading, one of my favorite pastimes, was suddenly challenging to the point of impossible. Print worsened my headaches. I couldn't focus or remember what I'd just read.

Family gatherings, once a source of comfort and connection, became painful and overwhelming. I couldn't follow group conversations or remember what people told me. I spoke slowly and haltingly. Sometimes I lost my words altogether. Often, I didn't speak at all.

I felt so alone, like a stranger among the people who knew me best. It was like I'd lost my place in my own family. As a grown-up, independent woman, I was embarrassed by how much assistance I needed from my family and friends. I often called them in tears, confused and uncertain what to do. I desperately needed their help, but often didn't want to accept it. I felt like a burden, a failure, and an adult who could no longer function.

My emotions were intense and unpredictable. I sobbed uncontrollably during sappy television commercials, melted down whenever plans changed unexpectedly, and slid down the wall crying when a bumblebee flew into my house. I thought I was losing my mind.

I kept trying to push through, believing hard work could fix anything. But the harder I tried, the worse everything got. I blamed myself for being weak, for being lazy, and for not trying hard enough. None of those harsh judgements were true, but I couldn't see that yet.

I tried and failed, over and over, to return to teaching. I tried and failed, over and over, to return to music. Eventually, I had to let go of both. My life shrank to medical appointments and four naps a day. I didn't recognize myself anymore. The identity I'd cherished as the *brain* was gone. Every day was a struggle just to function.

As the magnitude of the losses became clear, grief set in. I wasn't just grieving what I'd lost; I was grieving who I'd lost. The old Carole was gone. The new Carole felt like a stranger, one I didn't want to know. The grief was more intense than any I'd felt before. It was even greater than the grief of losing loved ones. This time, I was the one who had died.

There were many dark moments when I didn't think I could go on. Many times when I contemplated ending my life. But I didn't. And I'm deeply grateful I didn't.

It took me eight years and much help from professionals, family, friends, and other brain injury survivors to come to terms with this new version of myself. Accepting my life as a brain injury survivor was the hardest thing I've ever done. My first book, *To Root & To Rise: Accepting Brain Injury,* traces that journey toward acceptance.

I thought I lost what defined me—my intellect, teaching, music. But I didn't. Those parts of me aren't gone, but rather transformed. Music lives in the cadence of my writing. I now teach as a brain injury author, speaker, group leader, and mentor. My new self is still smart and driven, but also more balanced with increased empathy, perception, and wisdom.

I cope with daily brain injury symptoms, and my life is very different than I imagined. But it is a life filled with meaning, purpose, and joy.

As of this writing, I've been living with brain injury for twenty-five years. It's time to reflect and share what I've learned. Because even though this journey has brought grief and struggle, it has also led to unexpected joys and discoveries.

The lessons in this book come from my lived experience. I am not a medical or mental health professional. I am a brain injury survivor sharing what I've learned with others walking this path. Take what's helpful. Leave the rest.

Let's begin.

INTRODUCTION

Silver Threads

July 6ᵗʰ, 1999, the day of my brain injury, was a defining milestone.

July 6ᵗʰ, 2024 marked another milestone. My silver anniversary. Twenty-five years of living with brain injury.

Twenty-five years is a long time. Long enough to grieve and to find joy again. Long enough to struggle, to grow, and to gather wisdom. Long enough to discover that living well with brain injury isn't about returning to who I was; it's about becoming who I am now.

So, in honor of my twenty-five years, I'm sharing twenty-five lessons about living with brain injury—silver threads drawn from the fabric of my journey. These lessons began as a conference speech. Now I've expanded them into this book.

These silver learnings offer valuable insights, tested strategies, and practical wisdom with relevance for brain injury survivors, caregivers, and professionals.

The twenty-five lessons are grouped into five categories:

- Coping with Brain Injury
- Hard Truths
- Helpful Mindsets
- Accepting a New Self
- Thriving with Brain Injury

These categories not only help you navigate this book. They also reflect the broader process of navigating change, especially the kind we never asked for or expected.

Brain injury is a milestone that changes not only the direction of our lives, but more deeply, who we are as people. In the face of that unwelcome change, we gradually learn strategies to cope. We come face-to-face with hard truths we wish we could avoid. We discover that how we think—about ourselves, our injury, and our path forward—matters. And even though it may seem impossible at first, we begin to understand it is possible to come to terms with a changed life and to slowly build a meaningful new one.

This process doesn't move in a straight line; it is a spiral path that twists and turns. Sometimes we move forward, sometimes we loop backward, and sometimes we stand still. The lessons in this book honor that spiral path.

The brain injury journey will be different for each of us. These lessons are meant to meet you wherever you are on your path, offering encouragement, insight, and support as you navigate your way forward.

If you're a brain injury survivor reading this, I hope these hard-won lessons speak to your experience and help make the path ahead a little easier.

If you're a caregiver, I hope these lessons provide a window into pieces of your loved one's journey and open the door to meaningful conversations.

If you're a brain injury professional, I hope these lessons offer survivor-earned wisdom you can carry into your work, complementing your clinical knowledge and care.

However you engage with this book, I hope you find strength, meaning, and hope within it.

How to Read Silver Learnings

This book is written and formatted with brain injury survivors in mind. Paragraphs and chapters are short, since it can be hard to focus on long stretches of text. The print is larger than average, with extra spaces between paragraphs, to help reduce the overwhelmed feeling that reading can sometimes bring. I made these design choices to help make this book more accessible for brain injury survivors.

Each chapter stands on its own, so you can read them in any order. Choose the lessons most meaningful to you. This format also honors the memory challenges that many of us cope with. You don't need to remember earlier chapters to understand later ones. I designed this book to be flexible, so you can use it in whatever way best supports your journey.

At the end of each chapter, you'll find individual questions and an action item to help you reflect, explore, and apply the key ideas from the lesson to your own experience. There are also group discussion questions designed for brain injury support groups.

Silver Learnings is not a book of easy answers or quick solutions, because brain injury doesn't work that way.

But it <u>is</u> a book of hope. A book of wisdom. A book of practical advice from someone who has lived the journey.

Wherever you are on this path, I am honored to walk alongside you, and I hope my silver learnings inspire you to gradually notice and gather your own.

SECTION ONE:

COPING WITH BRAIN INJURY

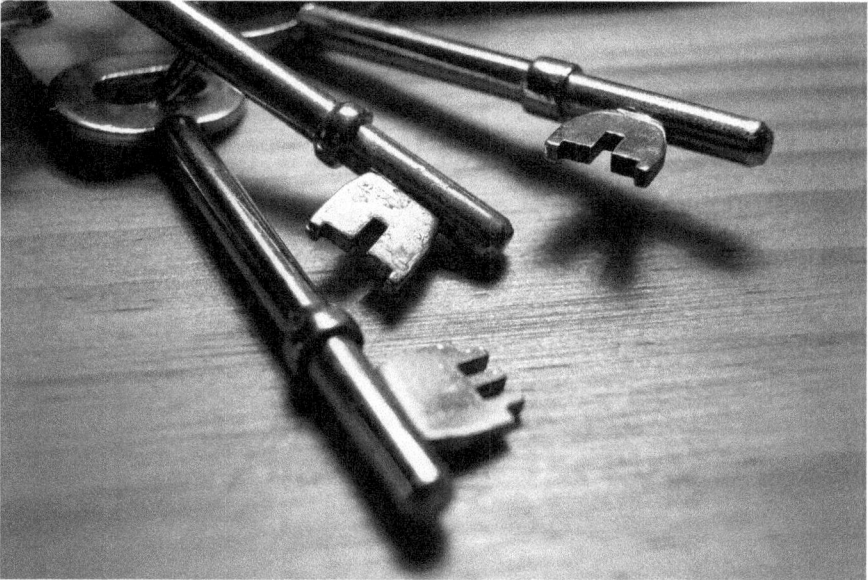

As we navigate our way through the early months and years after brain injury, it can feel like every way we turn, we face closed doors. Return to old life—door closed. Return to old self—door closed. Return to brain functioning as it always had—door closed.

That's a lot of doors closed in our face. We need keys. Keys to cope with the changes brain injury brings. Keys to unlock the doors to our new lives.

Coping with brain injury is about learning to recognize and deal with what is. Coping is about finding ways to handle the many symptoms we live with and the daily challenges we face.

The following five lessons have been key for me in learning to successfully cope with brain injury. These lessons were key at the beginning of my journey, and they are key now, twenty-five years later.

- Be willing to try a variety of treatment modalities
- Embrace strategies: Use what works now
- Learn when to push and when to pace
- Get to know your new self: What are your brain injury's tells?
- Know that sometimes your brain will lie to you

These lessons aren't keys that can open the doors leading back to our old lives and selves. For many of us, those doors are locked forever. Instead, these lessons are keys that can open doors to learning to cope with brain injury and to living our new lives.

1.

Be Willing to Try a
Variety of Treatment Modalities

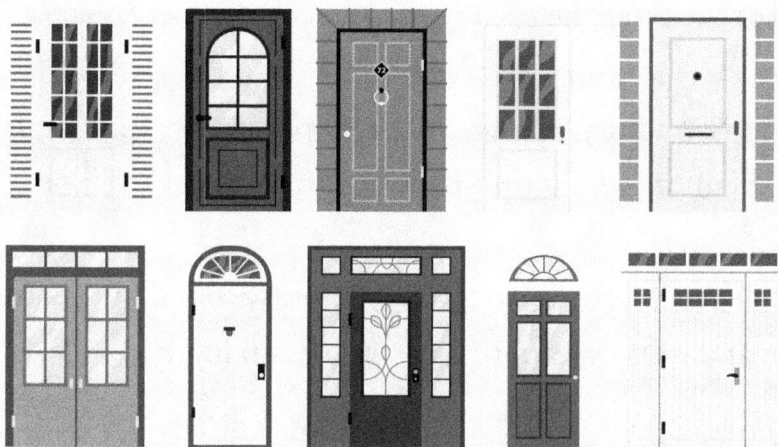

Sensvector/Shutterstock.com

This lesson may sound basic at first: *Be willing to try a variety of treatment modalities*. But in reality, this lesson is foundational to learning to cope with brain injury.

Brain injury can shatter us in multiple dimensions. We can get torn apart mentally, physically, emotionally, and spiritually.

Coping with brain injury means learning how to piece ourselves back together and finding our own individual path toward wholeness and a new life.

To do that, we need help, usually lots of it. There is no one person or treatment with all the answers that can put our pieces back together.

The brain injury journey is one of passing through multiple doors, of trying multiple treatment modalities.

Each door we pass through can help us rebuild our shattered lives and help us learn to cope with brain injury.

Because every person is different and every brain injury is different, it's difficult to predict the impact of any particular treatment.

What we <u>can</u> do is resolve to try and give it our best. We can choose to believe in the power of time, effort, and persistence to move us forward.

It's true no treatment has cured me; I still live with daily brain injury symptoms and will for the rest of my life. However, even tiny improvements have made a large difference in my day-to-day life.

To show just how varied this journey can be, here's an alphabetical list of the modalities I've tried over the years. Some are well-known and some are more unconventional. Each one is a door I chose to open.

Audiology	Neuropsychology
BodyTalk	Occupational Therapy
Counseling	Osteopathy
Craniosacral	Peer Counseling
Ear/Nose/Throat	Physiatry
Homeopathy	Physical Therapy
Massage	Social Work
Neurology	Speech Therapy
NeuroOptometry	Therapeutic Recreation
Neuropsychiatry	

This list is far from comprehensive. There are many more treatment options out there.

Some of these modalities worked great for me, while others did nothing. A few even set me back temporarily. Treatments varied from short-term to long-term ones that I continue to this day.

I'm purposefully not offering specific details. As I mentioned earlier, every person and every brain injury is unique, which means my experience may not be true for others.

I don't regret trying any of these modalities, even the ones that set me back for a while. A variety of treatments provide more than opportunities to heal. They also provide opportunities to learn about our brain injuries, to learn about ourselves, to develop self-advocacy skills, and to increase our resilience. All of that is part of coping with brain injury.

With that said, trying multiple treatment modalities has presented some challenges. There have been times in my journey, especially in the early years, when I felt like a professional patient. My days consisted mostly of medical appointments and resting to recover from medical appointments.

I've learned the hard way that more is not always better when it comes to treatment. The phrase *too many cooks in the kitchen* applies to brain injury. Too many modalities at the same time can lead to overload. Knowing when to say no and take a break can be just as important as being open to trying something new.

I've also learned that being open doesn't mean trying everything. Some treatments may carry risks or be a poor fit for our particular injuries. It's important to stay informed, trust our instincts, and ask for help from trusted advisors. If something doesn't feel right, it's okay to say no.

How does one find a variety of treatment modalities? I am not a medical professional, and had no idea what therapies I needed after my brain injury. I'd never heard of most of the modalities I've tried.

Like everything with brain injury, it's a process. We can learn about possibilities through recommendations from medical providers, by reading brain injury books, by talking to other brain injury survivors, and from attending brain injury conferences. Developing a trusted team is a strategy to help us in deciding which treatments to try.

Brain injury may close the door to our old lives, but trying new treatment modalities is a key that can open new doors to healing, growth, and new possibilities.

Making It Your Own: Applying Silver Learnings

This section offers space to reflect on how you've approached brain injury treatments. The questions and action item below are designed to help you connect your experience to the key ideas from this lesson: deciding which treatments to try, learning from what helped or didn't, and knowing when to take a break.

Section 1: Individual Reflection Questions

- How open have I been to trying different treatments or therapies?

- What's one treatment I tried that taught me something about myself or my brain injury?

- Have I ever felt like I was doing too many treatments at once?

Section 2: Group Discussion Questions

- How do you find out about new treatment options? What sources do you trust the most?

- Have you ever experienced a setback from a treatment? How did you cope and what did you learn?

- Is there a treatment modality you've been curious about but haven't tried yet? What's holding you back?

Section 3: Action Item—Suggestion for a Next Step after Reading Lesson 1

- Find Your Next Doorway

  o Write down one or two treatment modalities or therapies you've heard about but haven't tried yet. Use the list on page 25 if you need some ideas.

  o Talk with a trusted medical provider, family member, friend or fellow brain injury survivor about whether one of these might be worth exploring for your own healing journey.

2.

Embrace Strategies: Use What Works Now

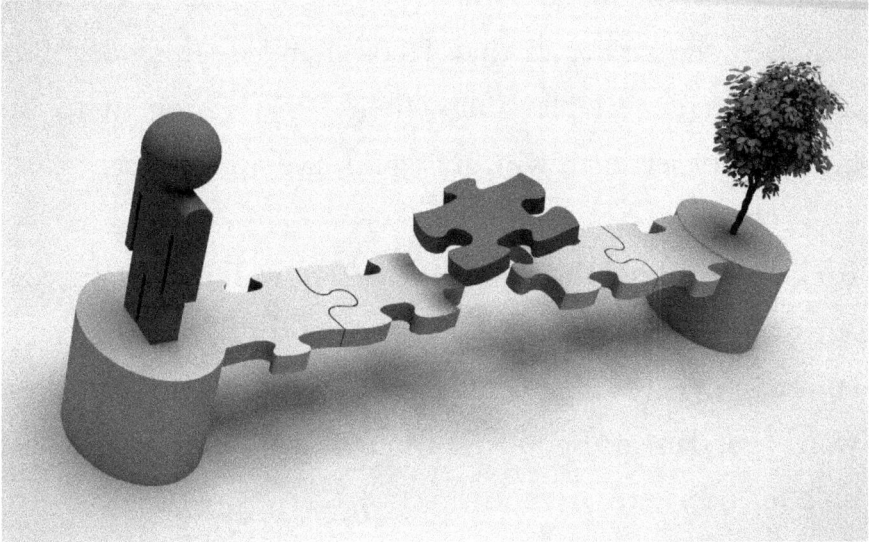

In the first year after my brain injury, I was confused, lost, isolated, and afraid. I kept trying to return to my old life, only to fail repeatedly. When I was eventually referred to an outpatient brain injury rehabilitation program, I was relieved. Finally, someone was going to fix me so I could get back to my life!

When the rehabilitation program began, I was surprised and dismayed that my therapists focused much of our time together talking about how I could compensate for my challenges by using strategies. They wanted me to learn to manage my brain injury deficits. I wanted them to make those deficits disappear and heal my brain injury.

I resisted my therapist's strategy-based approach. I believed if I used the strategies they recommended—memory aids, lists, pacing, meal planning—then I was giving in to the brain injury, letting it win, giving up, and not healing.

Back to my pre-injury normal was how I judged success. Anything that didn't measure up to that standard was a failure in my eyes. If I couldn't get back to who I was, I was worthless, damaged goods. I thought using strategies would hold me back.

I was wrong in how I looked at strategies. Accepting and using them don't hold us back. Strategies can help move us forward. They're not a roadblock to progress; they're a bridge to a new life.

Strategies can help us build a path to success. When there is a space between where we are now and where we want to be, strategies can be the missing puzzle piece that fills in the gap.

Strategies keep us focused on the present. When we concentrate on who we are now and embrace what works for us in this moment, we set ourselves up for a better life.

One of my biggest fears was that using strategies would stop my brain from healing. That hasn't been true for me. I use strategies, and I continue to make small gains to this day.

I've learned that pursuing healing and using strategies are not mutually exclusive. We don't have to choose one over the other. Both can happen together, and both can help us move forward.

Many of us start out resistant to using strategies. For a long time, all we can see is getting back to the lives we had. It takes time to recognize what's been lost and to grieve. Overcoming resistance is a process.

I can't say I let go of resistance and embraced strategies because I saw the logic in using them. Family, friends, and brain injury professionals were all unsuccessful in convincing me. I know my resistance frustrated them at times.

When I did eventually embrace strategies, it was mostly due to a combination of exhaustion and inspiration. Failing repeatedly at previously simple tasks wore me down. Those failures brought on exhaustion and a desperate desire to succeed again. That softened my resistance and opened me up to trying strategies to manage my life.

The inspiration came from other brain injury survivors. Through the outpatient brain injury rehabilitation program I attended, I met brain injury survivors whose injuries were older than mine. They modeled using strategies to make their lives work better. The example of my peers got through to me when no one else could.

Now, as a whole-hearted strategy embracer, whenever a task is difficult or I get overwhelmed, my first thoughts are, *What strategy can I use?* or *Who can help me figure out a strategy that will help?*

That enthusiasm comes with a disclaimer. Even now, as someone who uses strategies, I still sometimes feel stabs of sadness. There are moments I miss the old Carole and the ease of how things used to be. I wish I didn't need strategies. That ongoing grief is also part of the brain injury journey.

However, there is no question that using strategies has made my life better. Embracing strategies can give us feelings of success instead of failure, help us live in the now rather than getting lost in the past, make life easier, and preserve our energy for other tasks.

Strategies are not signs of defeat. They are signs of adaptation, creativity, and strength. Using them is a key to coping with brain injury.

Making It Your Own: Applying Silver Learnings

Here's an opportunity to reflect on your progress and challenges with strategies. The questions and action item below are designed to help you connect your experience to the key ideas from this lesson: letting go of returning to the way life used to be, seeing strategies as strengths, overcoming resistance, and learning from peers.

Section 1: Individual Reflection Questions

- Have I been resistant to using strategies because I wanted to do tasks the way I used to?

- Who could help me if I feel uncertain about using strategies?

- How do I feel when a strategy works well, even if it's different from how I used to do things?

Section 2: Group Discussion Questions

- How has your view of strategies changed over time? Do you see using strategies as a sign of strength, as a weakness, or as something else?

- What specific strategies have worked best for you in your daily life?

- What advice would you have for another brain injury survivor who feels resistant to using strategies?

Section 3: Action Item—Suggestion for a Next Step after Reading Lesson 2

- Choose & Use a Strategy

  o Pick one task in your life that feels difficult right now.

  o Brainstorm a new strategy (on your own or with someone you trust) that might help with that task.

  o Try the strategy out.

  o Afterwards, reflect on how the strategy worked.
    - Do you need to adjust the strategy?
    - Do you want to try a different strategy?

3.

Learn When to Push and When to Pace

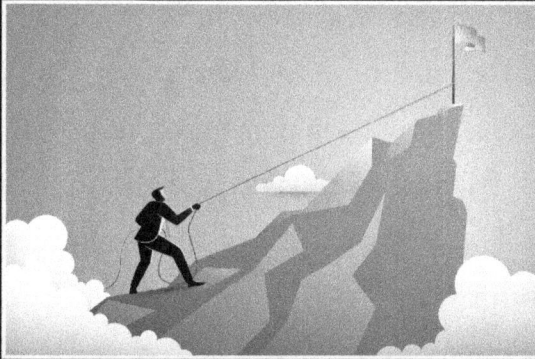

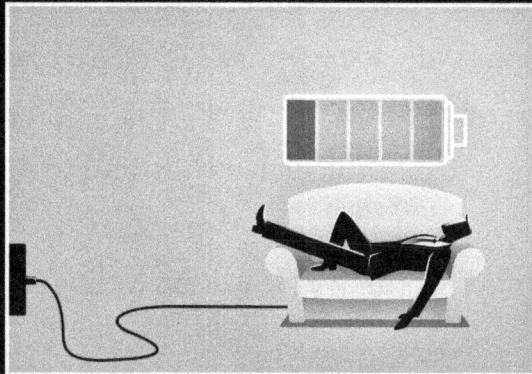

There are times in our brain injury journey when we have to push, because there's a mountain ahead for us to climb. Then, there are times when we need to pace, in order to recover from climbing that mountain.

Coping with brain injury means walking a fine line between pushing and pacing. Both are important tools for managing our lives and our energy levels.

During the early months and years after brain injury, handling the basics of life can be a steep climb. We may need to relearn how to take care of ourselves, how to support ourselves or our families, how to manage tasks at home, and how to socialize with friends. We may spend a lot of time in a variety of medical settings. All of that requires an enormous amount of push.

The truth is, to move forward after brain injury, some pushing will be necessary. To recover as much as possible, it's important to do the work of rehabilitation, to attempt new things, to take calculated risks, and to push our boundaries.

In other words, we have to be willing to climb the mountain.

However, there is also a real danger in pushing too much, too hard, and too fast, in ways our brains can't tolerate. That leads to falling off the mountain.

Too much time spent pushing is a recipe for brain overwhelm and overload. It may take us hours, days, or weeks to recover our energy.

Emotionally, too much pushing can leave us feeling broken, bruised, and defeated. This has happened to me many times over the years.

That's why pacing is just as important as pushing.

Pace recognizes that rest and recovery are necessary to balance out push.

Pace offers us time for reflection. When we get to know our new selves, we learn how much we can do and what our brains can handle.

Pace encourages us to pay attention to our internal battery. It's important to stop before our energy is completely depleted, and we're exhausted and overwhelmed for days.

However, just as there is danger in spending too much time in push, there is also danger in spending too much time in pace.

Too much time in pace can lead to giving up, to stagnating, to not trying new things, to not leaving the house, to not taking risks, and to believing where we are now is where we will always be.

How can we balance push and pace?

Because I struggle with pacing, that's what I had to focus more on. For me, push takes care of itself; I always push. I often had trouble recognizing when to stop pushing. (I still do sometimes.)

My brain injury rehab therapists modeled pacing for me. One of the most profound examples occurred one day when I arrived at the brain injury program and found all my therapists waiting for me in the treatment room. They told me they were cancelling half my therapy schedule, because it was too much for my brain. I cried with relief. I had been struggling, but I didn't know what to do. I had been trying to push, when I needed to pace.

My therapists helped me learn to recognize the signs that I need to pace. These signs are still true for me today.

I need to pace when:
- activities I'm attempting tire me into the next day
- the meal planning and cooking strategies I've mastered fall apart
- I constantly feel pressure in my head
- I get confused a lot
- I cry easily over nothing

Knowing when to pace comes down to observation, which helps us get to know ourselves and our brains.

Knowing when to pace is also about structure.

It can be difficult for me to recognize when to pace, because my brain lies to me about how much I can do. Therefore, pacing is built into the structure of my life in a variety of ways.

I enter every activity on my schedule, including meal and rest times. That makes it less likely I'll overschedule myself.

I generally schedule one activity in the morning and one in the afternoon. I try to be out of the house either in the morning or in the afternoon.

If I know an activity will be extra brain tiring, it will be the only event on my schedule that day, because it's likely I will need to rest for the remainder of the day.

Every week, there are days in my schedule with nothing planned, to allow time for my brain to recover.

I use a 10-point brain scale to assess my fatigue throughout the day. When I'm a 5 on the scale, I've learned that even though my brain will be telling me to push, I am starting to struggle. I just don't realize it. My brain lies to me when I'm a 5 on the scale. Therefore, 5 means I stop and rest, even though I don't want to or think I need to.

Over the years, I've developed guidelines for how often I can do activities, based on how long it takes me to recover from them. For example, hosting a big holiday dinner takes me several days to a week to fully recover from. Therefore, I only host holidays occasionally. The recovery cost is too high for me to do a lot of them. In contrast, going out to lunch with friends generally tires me for a few hours afterward, so it's something I can do more often.

I've found when I pace well, my brain energy stays more consistent. My motto is, *It's not a race; it's a pace.*

All those strategies may make it seem like I've perfected pacing. I have not. I still have a brain injury, and I still sometimes overestimate what I can do.

Finding the balance between pushing and pacing is an ongoing challenge for all of us. It's easy to fall off the mountain from pushing too much or to languish too long on the couch from pacing too much. All we can do each day is our best, to continue to walk the tight rope, and to give ourselves grace when we stumble.

Making It Your Own: Applying Silver Learnings

Use this space to reflect on how you manage your energy after brain injury. The questions and action item below are designed to help you connect your experience to the key ideas from this lesson: knowing when to push or pace, recognizing patterns in activity levels, and using structure to keep daily life manageable.

Section 1: Individual Reflection Questions

- Do I tend to push too far or pace too long?

- What signs does my body or brain give me when I've pushed too far or paced too long?

- Who helps me notice when I've pushed or paced too much? Do I accept what they tell me?

Section 2: Group Discussion Questions

- What are some ways you challenge yourself during a day or week (pushing)?

- What are some ways you build rest and recovery into your schedule (pacing)?

- What are the consequences to your life when you push too much? When you pace too much?

Section 3: Action Item—Suggestion for a Next Step after Reading Lesson 3

- Try a Pacing Practice

  o Choose one small pacing strategy to test this week. Some possibilities could be:
    - Taking a short rest before you feel tired
    - Scheduling fewer activities in one day
    - Adding a day with nothing planned to your calendar

  o Try the strategy to see if it helps your brain feel more balanced or rested.

4.

Get to Know Your New Self:
What Are Your Brain Injury's Tells?

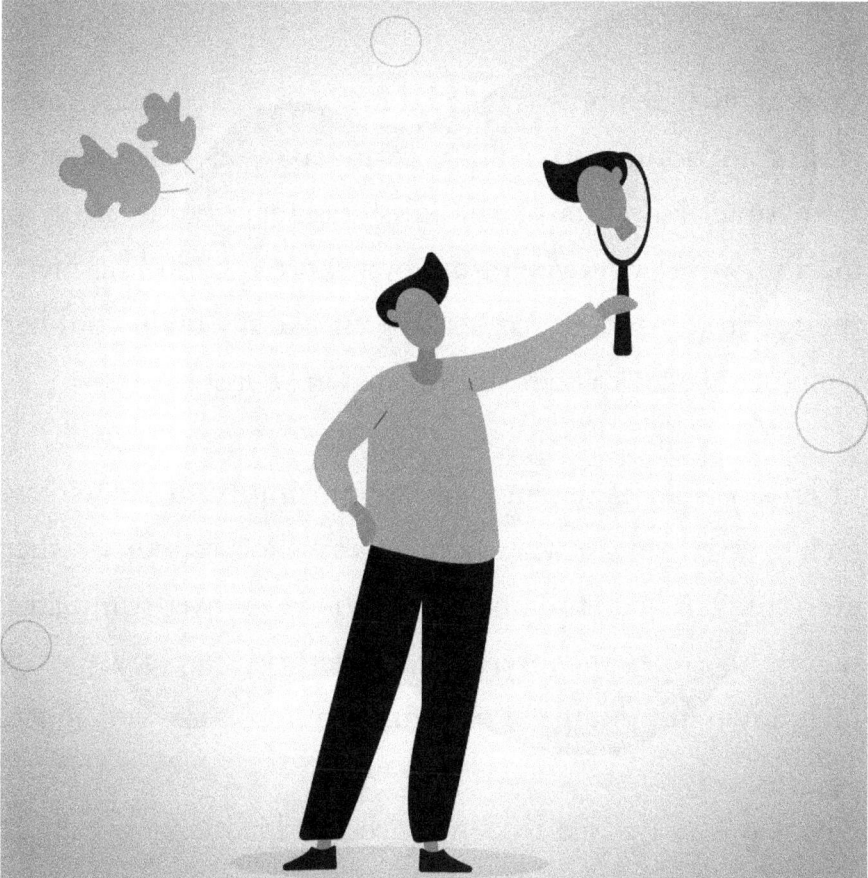

I like the graphic above, because it reminds me of my own early months and years after brain injury. Many times, I remember looking in the mirror and thinking that even though I looked like the same, pre-accident Carole, I didn't feel like the same Carole anymore. I would stare at my reflection and wonder, *Who are you?* I felt like I didn't recognize myself anymore. I hated the new person staring back at me in the mirror. I hated that brain injury had stolen my identity, turning me into someone I didn't want to be.

I especially hated how fragile I'd become, as I quickly tipped from functioning to failing, from engaged to exhausted. Even small amounts of thinking, talking, sound, light, or motion would overwhelm my brain, often confining me to the couch for days to recover. It felt like my brain could go from being okay to being overloaded in an instant.

Overload is an experience most brain injury survivors have had. Overload is when our brain short circuits, when everything is just too much, when we're over-stimulated, unable to cope, and overdone. Overload may cause us to melt down in a puddle of tears or erupt into a spew of anger.

The way I've learned to cope with overload is by getting to know my brain injury's tells. Just like a person playing poker has tells—body language indicating they're bluffing—our brain injuries have tells, signs indicating overload is building.

The trick is getting to know our new selves and learning to recognize those signs, so we can act and potentially stop (or at least reduce) overload before it's progressed too far.

Coping with brain injury means learning to be a good self-observer.

I am eternally grateful to my rehab therapists, other medical professionals, family, friends, and other brain injury survivors who helped me learn to observe and recognize my brain injury's tells. So much of what I know now started with the help of others. Learning to cope with brain injury is a team endeavor.

My journey learning to manage brain overload began with my team sharing their observations. They could see visible tells that my brain was going downhill.

Those tells included a dullness coming into my eyes and my expression changing. We called it my deer-in-the-headlights look. My brow would furrow as concentration grew more difficult. My speech would grow halting. I would lose my words more frequently and eventually stop talking all together. I would lose my balance more often. Tears flowed easily.

While knowing these tells was useful, by the time they were visible to others, I had already passed the point of no return. Overload was taking over and nearly impossible to stop.

To catch overload before it fully takes hold requires my internal observations. I had to learn to recognize the invisible tells that people can't see, but I feel.

The observations of my team taught me to trust my own. They helped me realize that the subtle signals I noticed— things no one else could see—meant something.

Here are some of my brain injury's internal tells, the signs of overload only I can notice:

Pressure in the left side of my head. It starts out subtle but will gradually get more pronounced, progressing to a desperate feeling that I need to lie down.

Labored speaking. To me, it feels like I'm talking through Jello or cotton. No one else will notice any change in my talking, but I know I'm struggling.

A general feeling that the world is going by too fast. No matter how slow the pace, I will feel like I'm struggling to keep up.

Difficulty with simple activities. I'll begin to mentally talk myself through how to do everyday tasks, such as getting dressed, making coffee, or cleaning the house.

Difficulty sequencing. I won't be able to follow anything that goes step by step, such as directions or a recipe.

Euphoria. Yes, euphoria. I've learned that not all tells feel bad at first. This one feels deceptively amazing. The euphoria happens when I'm feeling great. It happens when it's getting to be my normal rest time, and I still feel fine. Or I've just done something extra cognitive, but I'm not extra tired.

I experience a surge of euphoria, accompanied by the thought, *Today's the day! I don't need a nap!* It lasts 10-20 minutes, then my brain starts going downhill and the other tells appear as overload builds. The euphoria is my brain's version of a mirage, of false hope before the crash.

The trick to stopping overload is first recognizing the tells and then acting on them. If I stop, take a break, lie down and rest, or remove myself from the situation, then I have a chance to prevent overload from happening.

Recognizing and acting on my tells doesn't always work perfectly. Sometimes life happens fast, or brain injury symptoms come on too quickly, and overload happens anyway. Even if I can't fully stop overload, I may be able to lessen its impact and reduce how much time it takes me to recover.

There's so much about brain injury that is out of our hands. Getting to know our tells can give us back one small measure of control.

The better we know ourselves and the better we know our tells as brain injury survivors, the more choices we have. We can step away before we crash. We can rest before we unravel. Even during times when overload happens anyway, we can know we're doing our best. Knowledge and choices give us more power over our lives.

Socrates said, *To know thyself is the beginning of wisdom.* To know thyself is also the beginning of coping with brain injury.

Making It Your Own: Applying Silver Learnings

This reflection section is an opportunity to deepen your understanding of overload and brain injury tells. The questions and action item below are designed to help you connect your experience to the key ideas from this lesson: recognizing early signs of overload, taking action before symptoms get worse, and accepting help from others.

Section 1: Individual Reflection Questions

- When am I most likely to experience brain overload?

- What is one visible sign others might notice when overload is building in me?

- What is one subtle or invisible overload sign only I feel or notice?

Section 2: Group Discussion Questions

- What makes it difficult to notice your brain injury's tells?

- What could you do to reduce or even stop overload once you notice it building?

- Who are the people who could help you notice overload?

Section 3: Action Item—Suggestion for a Next Step after Reading Lesson 4

- Catch a Tell in Real Time

  o Over the next few days, watch for one of your brain injury's tells, a sign that overload is building. When you notice it, pause.

  o Name the tell to yourself (for example, *My words are slowing down,* or *I feel pressure in my head*).

  o Try a coping strategy immediately, such as resting, stepping away, dimming the lights, or reducing stimulation with earplugs, sunglasses, or a hat.

  o Later, ask yourself if the strategy helped prevent or reduce overload.

5.

Know That
Sometimes Your Brain Will Lie to You

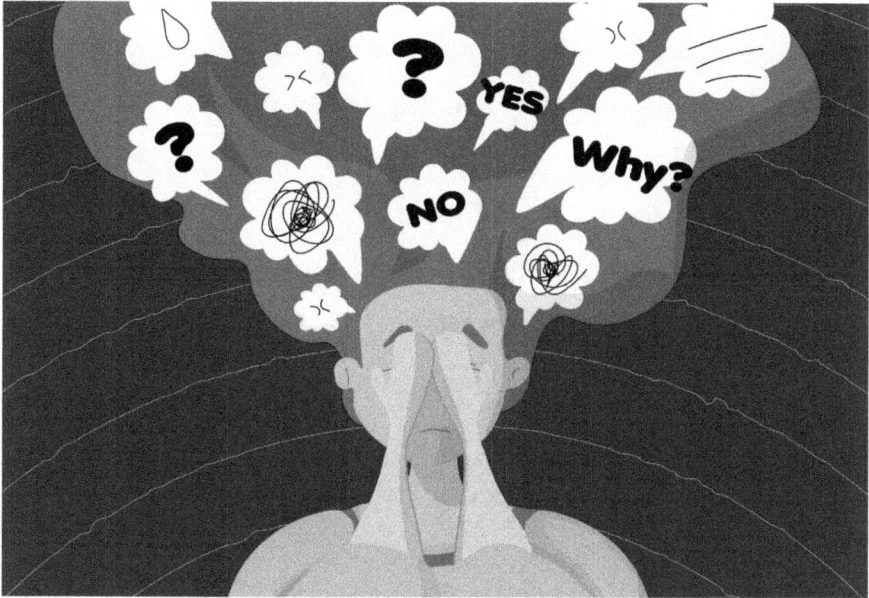

It is a frustrating truth of brain injury: our brains lie to us. These aren't conscious lies we choose to tell. They're lies that come from denial, from lack of awareness, from false memories, and from the injury itself.

The lies our brains tell can seem so believable. They influence our thoughts, feelings, and actions.

Here are some of the convincing—but untrue—statements my brain has tried to make me believe over the years:

- Just push harder and you'll make a full recovery
- Tomorrow you will wake up *normal*
- You're worthless if you can't achieve like old Carole did
- The only life worth living is the one you had before brain injury
- You're not strong enough to cope with brain injury
- You'll never accomplish anything again
- You don't need strategies
- Today is the day you don't need a nap
- You won't need help with this task
- Your sense of direction is right when it says go *this way*
- You can choose the correct size bowl to store leftovers from dinner (I'll explain more about this one shortly!)

I know those statements are not true now, but at various times over the last twenty-five years, I have believed all of them.

Believing my brain's lies has caused me great emotional distress.

Believing my brain's lies has led me to do more than I'm capable of, overload, and need to be rescued.

Believing my brain's lies has made life more difficult for my family and friends and has made me a challenging patient at times.

Believing my brain's lies has led to getting lost.

Believing my brain's lies has filled up my fridge with large bowls containing small amounts of leftovers.

How do we know what is true and what is a lie our brain is telling us?

Left to my own devices, I might still believe all those lies. Professionals, family, and friends have helped me to untangle what is truth and what is not. It's been a process learning if and when I can trust what my brain tells me.

But to this day, my brain still lies to me. That is the nature of brain injury.

I divide the lies into two broad categories. There are lies that can be conquered and lies that need to be managed.

The lies that have been conquered are the ones about who I am, my worth as a person, my personal resilience, and the nature of the brain injury recovery process.

Those lies have been conquered by bringing them to the surface to examine and reflect on them, and by learning more about brain injury.

I make that sound easy. It was not. It took years and years, hard work, many tears, and lots of professional help.

The lies that need to be managed are trickier, because they are ongoing due to the nature of brain injury. Even though I know they're not true, I can still get tripped up by them.

Here's a funny example—my leftovers.

I know my brain lies to me when choosing what size bowl for the leftovers. I always think the bigger bowl is the right one. I cannot stop that lie from happening. It's part of the damage to my brain.

Here's how I manage it. I know it's a lie, so I rely on past experience. My past experience tells me I always choose too big a bowl. So, I choose the next size down, even though everything in me says that's wrong.

When our brains lie, using our past experience to guide us can be a strategy.

Here's another, more consequential example of managing my brain injury's lies. I have a hard time judging how much I can do. I regularly overestimate what I'm capable of. I take one small success and try to make it into something bigger.

In the early days after brain injury, I would have a good half hour, excitedly call family and friends, and confidently declare I was ready to return to work full time. I would be confused and heartbroken by their strong disagreement.

Twenty-five years later, my brain still lies to me the same way. The circumstances may be different, but the overestimating what I can do lie is the same.

For example, prior to my brain injury, I regularly traveled by myself to visit friends or attend professional conferences. Now, whenever a travel opportunity comes up, my brain is convinced I'm ready to fly solo again.

My brain tells me I no longer need a friend traveling with me to assist with logistics, unexpected situations, and sudden brain injury symptoms. Since I've successfully managed a few short solo flights with someone meeting me, my brain believes I should also be able to handle longer trips with connecting flights alone.

The difference between now and the early days after brain injury, is I know my brain lies to me about what I can do. And I know that relying on the advice of others is a strategy to manage those lies. This strategy can also keep me safe.

Each time I've asked my trusted team of professionals, family members, and friends whether I should travel on my own, the answer has been an emphatic no. They also all laugh at first. These are not unkind laughs, but familiar laughs that come from years of dealing with this brain injury lie.

Even though there is still part of me that thinks I should try a solo trip, I listen to my team, and I trust their advice. Each time it has been the right advice.

I admit it's been humbling to realize that until I thought more deeply about this lesson, I was unaware of how much my brain still lies to me, even after twenty-five years.

That is life with brain injury. It is an ongoing journey of increasing our awareness and using that awareness to develop strategies to cope. Our brains may lie, but we can still find truths to move us forward.

Making It Your Own: Applying Silver Learnings

Here is a chance to consider how brain injury lies show up in your life. The questions and action item below are designed to help you connect your experience to the key ideas from this lesson: noticing when the brain gives inaccurate information, getting help to sort out what's true, and finding ways to manage brain injury lies.

Section 1: Individual Reflection Questions

- What is one lie your brain injury has told you?

- How has believing that lie affected you?

- What strategy (or person) can help you challenge or manage that lie?

Section 2: Group Discussion Questions

- How do you know the difference between the truth and a lie your brain injury is telling you?

- Who are the people in your life who help you separate truth from lies? Do you listen to their advice?

- What strategies have you tried to cope with the lies your brain injury tells you?

Section 3: Action Item—Suggestion for a Next Step after Reading Lesson 5

- Take a 10-Second Pause

    o Pay attention to moments when your brain tells you something that might not be true, such as, *I don't need to rest*, or *I can do one more thing.*

    o Take a 10-second pause before you act.

    o During the pause, ask yourself a simple question such as, *Has this gone well before?* or *Could my brain be lying to me right now?*

SECTION TWO:

HARD TRUTHS

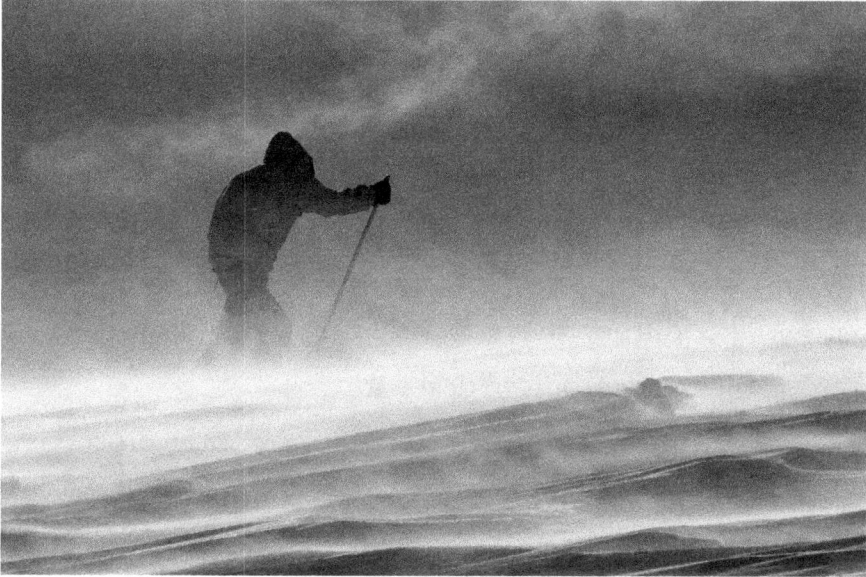

As we learn to cope with brain injury, we are going to run into hard truths, those harsh realities that come with a life-changing injury.

Icy winds, like those in the picture above, are a good metaphor for hard truths. Both are unwelcome and difficult to endure. They bring discomfort and pain. They can be unforgiving and relentless. They can leave us feeling vulnerable and disoriented.

Just as icy winds are part of nature, hard truths are part of life after brain injury. They cut through us, shatter illusions, and force us to confront realities we would rather not acknowledge.

Here are six hard truths I struggled with in my brain injury journey:

- The journey never ends: There will always be brain injury symptoms to deal with
- Learning to cope with failure is part of the process
- There will be many people who don't get it
- Feelings of grief and loss never completely go away
- Comparison is an ongoing struggle
- Even with strategies, expect your brain to be inconsistent

We face icy winds by dressing warmly and bracing against the cold. Similarly, we face brain injury hard truths by acknowledging them. We let ourselves feel what we feel. We reach out for support. We focus on what we can control and look for ways to learn and grow through the challenge.

Although these hard truths are difficult to face, they can also be catalysts for personal transformation. We may not be able to change the effects of brain injury on our lives, but confronting hard truths can strengthen our endurance, our wisdom, and our resilience.

6.

The Journey Never Ends: There Will Always Be Brain Injury Symptoms to Deal With

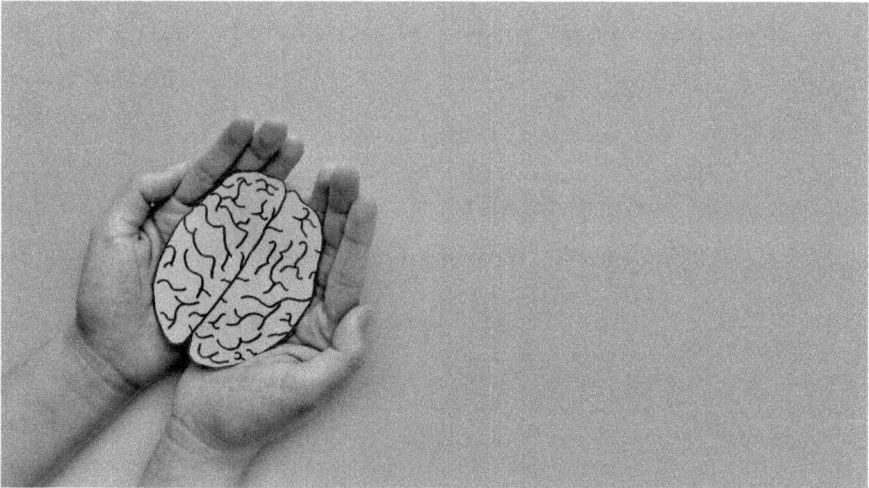

Orawan Pattarawimonchai/Shutterstock.com

For a long time, I thought that if I could just find the right treatments and strategies, then I would be able to control my brain injury and make it mostly disappear. I desperately wanted to be *normal* again. While I knew I couldn't make my brain injury completely go away, I thought that the right supports would make it invisible, both to me and the outside world. Wrong!

Let me first say there is no question that treatments and strategies can make life better after brain injury. I continue to work to improve my quality of life, and I continue to make progress.

However, even though I still see providers in a variety of modalities, and even though I use numerous strategies every day, I still have brain injury symptoms. My injury impacts my life every single day.

I can do everything right to manage my brain injury—use strategies, pace myself, honor my new self—but still there are days when my brain refuses to cooperate. Life falls apart, I overload, get confused, and I spend most of my time resting on the couch.

Dealing with ongoing symptoms and their fallout is part of the brain injury experience. I don't like it, but it is something to accept. It is a hard truth.

We get to be sad about hard truths. We get to be frustrated by them.

I freely admit that even though I have accepted all my *Silver Learning* hard truths, there are still times, all these years later, when I feel sad and frustrated by them.

And that's okay. By definition, hard truths challenge us. They are hard to accept, and they are hard to live with.

When we're confronted by the hard truth of ongoing brain injury symptoms, it's helpful to remember we do have choices. These choices remind us that we do have power.

We can choose to acknowledge the reality that brain injury has changed us forever.

We can choose to focus on living in the present moment, versus dwelling on the past, or worrying about the future.

We can choose to reach out for help when sadness or frustration well up.

We can choose to hold ourselves gently when brain injury symptoms rule our lives.

This chapter's image of a person cradling a brain speaks to the importance of treating ourselves with gentleness and care. Self-compassion can soften the sharp edges of hard truths and make them a little easier to live with.

The large amount of space around the brain in the picture matters too. We need both time and space to come to terms with the ongoing journey that is brain injury.

Space to absorb the hard truths.
Space to feel what we feel.
Space to breathe.
Space to rest.

There may always be brain injury symptoms to deal with, but we can choose to cradle ourselves gently and to honor whatever space we need to move forward.

Making It Your Own: Applying Silver Learnings

This section gives you space to reflect on the ongoing nature of brain injury. The questions and action item below are designed to help you connect your experience to the key ideas from this lesson: accepting that brain injury symptoms may continue, recognizing common responses when symptoms get worse, and practicing self-kindness on tough brain days.

Section 1: Individual Reflection Questions

- Have I been holding on to the hope of returning to my pre-brain injury life?

- When my brain injury symptoms increase, am I more likely to be hard on myself or to treat myself with compassion?

- What's one compassionate thing I can do for myself on a bad brain day?

Section 2: Group Discussion Questions

- Which brain injury symptoms are most difficult for you to accept?

- What helps you accept that brain injury is an ongoing journey?

- How do you show kindness to yourself when you're having a bad brain day?

Section 3: Action Item—Suggestion for a Next Step after Reading Lesson 6

- Create a Self-Compassion Cue

  o Choose a small object, photo, phrase, or quote that has meaning for you.

  o On bad brain days, hold, look at, or read the item you chose. Use it as a cue to remember to hold yourself gently, with kindness, and compassion.

7.

Learning to Cope with Failure
is Part of the Process

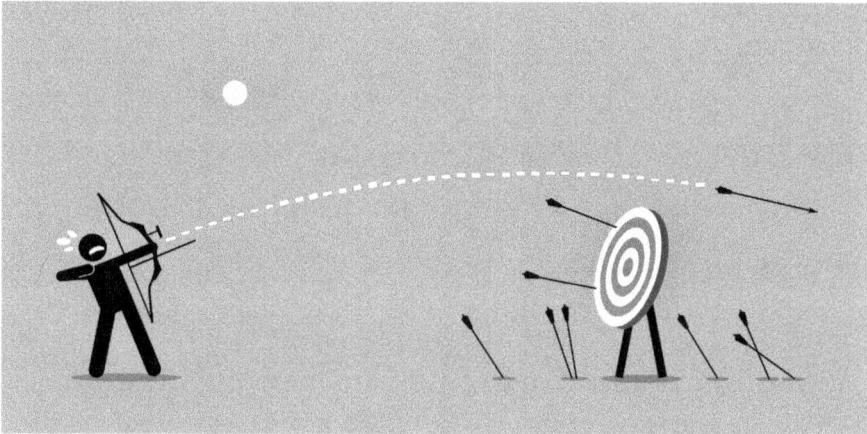

Failure. It's a harsh word, isn't it? I can almost hear some of you pushing back against my choice of that word.

When we're working hard to relearn old skills and build new lives, but sometimes miss the mark, wouldn't words like trying, effort, or practice be better words than failure?

Trying, effort, and practice are definitely more neutral and less emotionally loaded words than failure. But the truth is, when we repeatedly aim for and miss targets we used to hit easily, neutral words just don't describe the experience.

Failure is what it feels like on the inside. That's why that word is the focus of this lesson.

When I couldn't return to teaching and music, I felt like a failure. When I struggled to take care of myself, I felt like a failure. When family and friends had to rescue me, I felt like a failure.

Those feelings of failure decimated my self-esteem and self-confidence. I blamed myself for being weak and for not trying hard enough.

As you can probably tell, I was much too hard on myself. More than that, I was unfair to myself.

I wasn't failing due to a character defect. I wasn't lazy or unmotivated. The reality was I was failing because the tasks I kept attempting and the Carole I kept trying to be, were too much for my brain.

So, what can we do when we miss the mark? How can we cope with feelings of failure?

Here are two strategies that have been useful for me: Change the target and change the language. Both are about reframing failure.

If the target I'm aiming for is returning to life the way it was before my brain injury, I will fail. If the target I'm aiming for is trying to be old Carole, I will fail. So, I've had to change my targets.

Relearning how to plan and cook my meals is a good example of changing my targets. Before my brain injury, I would go to the grocery store, think about the meals I wanted to make for the week, walk the aisles, and purchase the necessary ingredients.

I didn't use a list, because I remembered what I needed and what I already had on hand at home. I was never a gourmet cook, but I could make tasty, nutritious meals without struggling.

After my brain injury, I tried to approach meal planning and cooking in the same relaxed way and failed. The noise, lights, motion, and visual clutter of the grocery store overloaded my brain the instant I walked in.

I couldn't think about what meals to make or remember what ingredients to buy. I got fixated on the idea of marinating meats and purchased sauces every week. But I couldn't make the meals, because I struggled to make decisions and follow a recipe. Eventually, I had an entire shelf full of unused marinades. Cottage cheese became my default dinner most nights.

Failing at a basic life task that had once been easy was embarrassing and demoralizing.

My occupational therapist helped me change the target by breaking meal planning and cooking down into smaller, more manageable pieces. These included a grocery list organized by aisle and a six-week rotating menu plan of simple meals I could make. My mom helped me make a list of emergency meals I could keep in the freezer. Changing the target to something doable helped me feel like a success, instead of like a failure.

Even when we've changed our target to something more doable, we can still miss the mark. Events happen that are out of our control.

Even though I now have well-honed strategies for meal planning and cooking, sometimes I still eat cottage cheese for dinner. I get busy and use up the mental energy I need to shop and cook. I forget about the emergency meals in the freezer. The grocery store is unexpectedly crowded, which leads to brain fatigue and confusion. Then, even though I have the ingredients to make a meal, I just can't.

That's why the second reframing failure strategy is important too. Change the language.

Change the language means when we miss the mark, we challenge any inner voice that says we're a failure. It means changing what we say to ourselves.

Statements like, *I'll never get this, I'm so stupid,* or *I always mess things up,* reinforce feelings of failure. Changing our language to statements such as, *I'm doing my best, Setbacks are part of the process, I'm making progress,* or *I'll take a nap and figure out what to do later,* help us shift from self-blame to self-support. These words remind us that although we may struggle, we are not failures.

The words we choose have power. When we choose to speak kindly to ourselves, we open ourselves to the learning and growth that can come from failures. We can become more resilient.

Living with brain injury means sometimes, as hard as we try, we will miss the mark. There will be failures, both large and small, to cope with. We may not be able to change that, but we can reframe those failures and learn from them.

Making It Your Own: Applying Silver Learnings

Here's a chance to pause and explore the topic of failure. The questions and action item below are designed to help you connect your experience to the key ideas from this lesson: noticing emotional reactions to failure, adjusting goals after setbacks, and using kinder language instead of self-criticism.

Section 1: Individual Reflection Questions

- What is one thing I tried to do recently where I missed the mark, and it didn't go how I had hoped?

- What did I tell myself when I missed the mark? Was I critical or kind when talking to myself?

- What is something I was able to complete by taking it step by step?

Section 2: Group Discussion Questions

- What does the word failure mean to you at this point in your journey?

- What does the phrase *adjust the target* mean to you? Can you think of a time when you did that?

- What have you realized or learned from failure?

Section 3: Action Item—Suggestion for a Next Step after Reading Lesson 7

- Snap & Shift

  o When you catch yourself thinking something harsh or critical about yourself such as, *I'm so stupid* or *I'll never get this*, snap your fingers.

  o Take a breath and change your language to something kind or neutral such as, *Try again, Take it step by step,* or *I'm doing the best I can.*

8.

There Will Be Many People Who Don't Get It

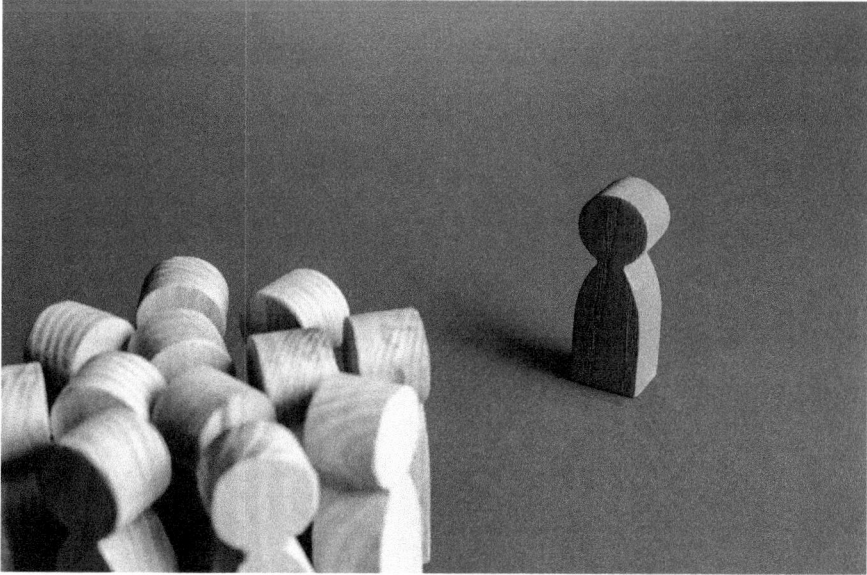

Andrii Yalanskyi/Shutterstock.com

Have you heard comments like these?

- You look fine
- You don't look like you have a brain injury
- Oh, that happens to me too
- Everyone forgets things
- It could have been worse
- You look great!
- Maybe you're just depressed...or anxious

- You're using your brain injury as an excuse
- You talk about your brain injury too much
- I wish I could take a nap every day

These aren't just harmless remarks. Whether they're said intentionally or unintentionally, these statements deny, dismiss, or distort our lived experience—and they hurt.

Every one of these comments have been said to me over the years, bringing on feelings of sadness, devastation, fear, anger, frustration, resignation, hopelessness, and now, even mild amusement.

It is an unfortunate reality that when an injury is mostly invisible and hard for people to understand, like brain injury is, then people will make comments that are ignorant, unthinking, unhelpful, and often hurtful.

The picture opening this chapter depicts how these comments can affect us. We may feel alone, like an outsider, or an *other*.

Early on in my brain injury journey, I thought the solution was getting people to stop saying hurtful comments. I thought if I just explained brain injury more, or if I explained the impact of the comments on me, then they would stop.

Sometimes explaining helped—but often, it didn't. I've come to accept that some people simply don't get it. There will always be hurtful comments.

I wish I could wave a magic wand and make others understand brain injury and realize the impact of their words. However, what other people say is out of our control.

What is in our control is how we react and how we feel about ourselves. I've found the stronger my new self became, the less other's words bothered me. Comments bounce off me easier now and are less likely to bring on strong emotions. After twenty-five years, they're more likely to amuse me at this point.

A strong sense of self is like a chainmail suit of armor. It's strong enough to deflect the hurt, but flexible enough to allow in the amusement.

So, how does one build that strong sense of self after brain injury? It's not a matter of *do this one thing* and poof—an instant strong self and chainmail suit of armor.

Instead, like everything with brain injury, building a strong sense of self takes time. It is an ongoing process, helped by family, friends, professionals, and other brain injury survivors.

Many of the *Silver Learning* lessons can help. I think of them as strands weaving together to create that chainmail suit. Get to know your new self. Find something the new you is good at. Connect with others who share the journey. Find humor. Own who you are. Assemble a team. Connect to your purpose. All of these are integral to building a strong sense of self.

Another strategy for coping with words that hurt is to choose our response. When confronted with people who don't get it, our actions are up to us. This does take practice. A good first step is to take a breath.

We may choose to protect ourselves. We can walk away or not engage, especially if it's clear that nothing we say will make a difference.

We may choose to educate. We can share our brain injury stories, correct misinformation, and explain why comments are hurtful.

We may choose to advocate. We can use our voices to make a difference for others.

No one response is better than the other. It's about where we are in our journey and the situation on any particular day. The choice is up to us.

There may be many people who don't get brain injury, but we are <u>not</u> powerless against what they say, and we are <u>not</u> alone.

Making It Your Own: Applying Silver Learnings

Use this section to reflect on how you deal with people who don't understand brain injury. The questions and action item below are designed to help you connect your experience to the key ideas from this lesson: recognizing the impact of hurtful comments, finding ways to stay strong, and choosing how to respond when someone says something hurtful.

Section 1: Individual Reflection Questions

- How do I feel when people don't understand my brain injury?

- What is one comment someone made that bothered me?

- What helps me stay strong, even when others don't understand my brain injury?

Section 2: Group Discussion Questions

- What comments have been hardest for you to hear?

- How do you decide whether or not to respond to hurtful comments?

- Has your reaction to comments changed over time? How so?

Section 3: Action Item—Suggestion for a Next Step after Reading Lesson 8

- Practice Responding to Hurtful Comments

  o Brainstorm (alone or with others) one thing you can say to protect yourself when someone says something hurtful (for example, *I'm going to leave this conversation now*).

  o Brainstorm one thing you can say to educate or advocate, if you choose to (for example, *Brain injury may be invisible, but it is real*).

  o Choose a way to stay calm (for example, *take a deep breath* or say to yourself, *I know what's true*).

  o Practice your responses with a trusted friend or family member.

9.

Feelings of Grief and Loss
Never Completely Go Away

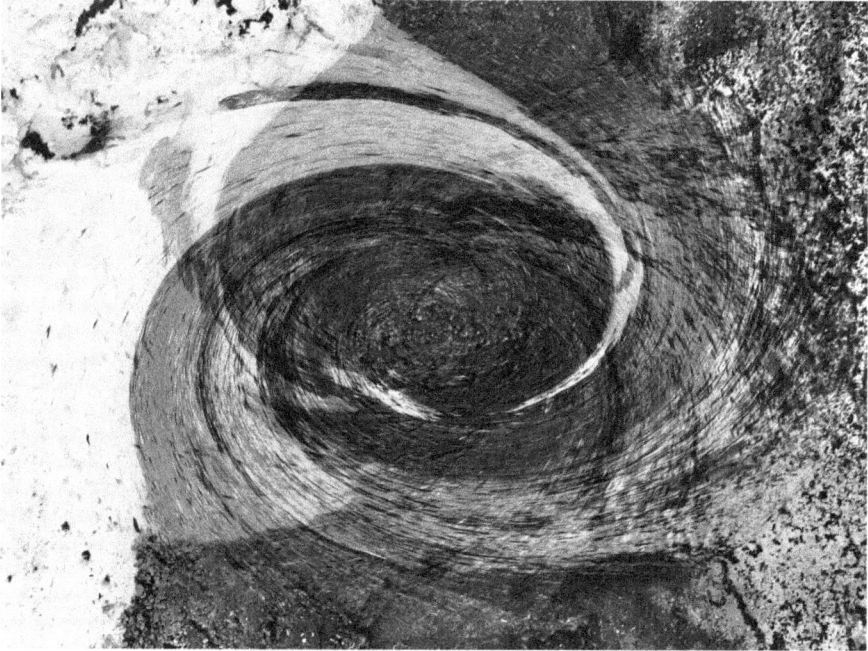

If you've ever lost someone you cherished, then you know the gaping hole that is grief. You've navigated the swirling tides of loss, trying to stay afloat.

At first after loss, that hole in our lives can feel all-consuming. With time, support from others, care, and compassion, grief can heal. That gaping hole can shrink as we learn to move forward without our loved one and as we accept a changed life.

But if you've grieved, you also know that although the gaping hole can narrow, it never goes away. We will always miss the one we loved.

Even when we've moved into a different life, there will be times when grief gets triggered—their birthday, an anniversary, hearing a song, seeing a picture, or thinking about a memory. That is the up and down, waxing and waning nature of loss.

After brain injury, we face a different kind of death—the death of the person we were, the life we lived, and the future we expected. All that loss triggers a profound grieving process.

I can honestly say brain injury grief was the worst grief I've ever felt. It was worse than the grief I experienced after my mother died. This time I was the one who died. My body may have been alive, but the self I knew was gone.

I mourned my lost self and shattered life for years. There were days when I thought the grief would swallow me whole, that I wasn't strong enough to make it through.

It took a long time and a lot of help from many people for my own gaping hole of grief after brain injury to shrink. But it did shrink. When we're grieving so much loss, getting help with the process can make a big difference.

Ever so slowly, I moved through denial, came to terms with the fact that my old life was over, learned to like myself again, found activities the new me could do, built community, and discovered a different purpose. Over time, I stopped defining myself by what I had lost.

Working through grief and loss after my brain injury has increased my empathy, perception, wisdom, and resilience. I am grateful for those gifts.

However, even though I've built a new life after brain injury and healed from the worst of my grief, there are still times when the loss hits me. I miss the Carole who died on July 6th, 1999. That hole is still there. It will always be there. And I've come to realize that's okay.

This lesson isn't about trying to erase the hole. It's about acknowledging and learning to manage it, so we don't get sucked in and overwhelmed.

All of us have triggers for our brain injury grief, which sometimes hit suddenly. Here are a few of mine; maybe some will be familiar to you too.

- Tasks that used to be easy but are now difficult
- Reminders of my old life
- A string of bad brain days with increased symptoms
- Having to give up something because of brain injury
- A reminder that tasks I struggle with are easy for other people

These triggers hurt, but not as much as they did when I was actively grieving. They're now more an echo of the sharper pain I felt earlier on.

What can we do when feelings of grief and loss hit?

Acknowledge the feelings. Don't try to cover them up with false positivity. That's a recipe for staying stuck in grief and loss. We get to feel sad sometimes. Brain injury is an all-consuming challenge. There's no question about it.

Develop strategies to cope. Strategies can help us avoid getting sucked into a whirlpool of grief. Strategies may include talking to professionals, family, friends, or other brain injury survivors, writing about our feelings, making art, spending time in nature, exercising, or meditating. It's about whatever helps. It's often a process to figure out what works for us as individuals.

When feelings of grief and loss hit me, my strategies are usually talking to other survivors, writing, and taking a walk. The combination of those three activities helps to validate my experience and work through my feelings, so I can return to this new life I lead.

These strategies can't erase the hole, but they do help manage it. This hard truth reminds us that although grief can heal, it still leaves a scar.

Making It Your Own: Applying Silver Learnings

This reflection section invites you to think about your own experience with brain injury grief. The questions and action item below are designed to help you connect your experience to the key ideas from this lesson: grieving our old selves is normal and necessary, grief shrinks but never fully goes away, and facing grief is a key to moving forward.

Section 1: Individual Reflection Questions

- What moments or situations tend to bring out my brain injury grief?

- What happens to me mentally, physically, and emotionally when my brain injury grief is triggered?

- Is there anything about my brain injury grief that's changed over time? If yes, what's changed?

Section 2: Group Discussion Questions

- What are some ways you manage your brain injury grief when it hits?

- What has grieving taught you about yourself?

- What would you say to someone who feels like their brain injury grief will never get better?

Section 3: Action Item—Suggestion for a Next Step after Reading Lesson 9

- Take a Comfort Break

  o When feelings of grief hit, give yourself permission to take a break and take care of yourself.

  o Do one small, comforting thing. For example:
    - Take a few deep breaths
    - Go outside
    - Listen to favorite music
    - Hold a treasured object
    - Look at a favorite picture
    - Write or draw in a journal
    - Call a trusted friend, family member, or professional

10.

Comparison is an Ongoing Struggle

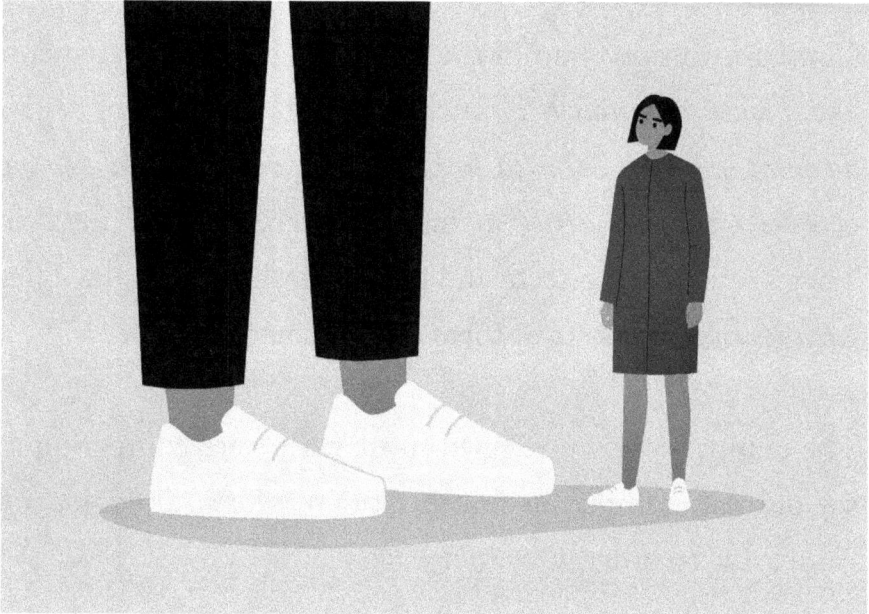

Comparison is a common trap to fall into. It can creep into our thoughts without us even realizing it, whispering that we're not good enough, smart enough, strong enough. Theodore Roosevelt summed it up well: *Comparison is the thief of joy.*

After brain injury, those whispers can turn into shouts as we compare ourselves endlessly—to our old selves, to other survivors, to impossible standards, to people without brain injuries. These comparisons can leave us feeling defeated and less than. The picture on the previous page captures the experience of the *other* looming large while we shrink in comparison.

Comparison shows up in the words we choose. Statements like, *I used to be able to do that task better/faster, Why can't I do what they do?, I should be healed by now*, or *I'm worth less because my life is different* make us feel small and inferior. They decrease self-esteem and increase feelings of guilt. They steal joy because none of them are fair comparisons.

The comparisons I struggled most with were comparing to my old self, comparing to other brain injury survivors, and comparing to other women my age.

If I compare myself to old Carole, I will always lose. As much as I've accomplished since my brain injury, I still can't hold a candle to her. Old Carole could work a full-time job during the day and then go to music rehearsals or social activities at night. I can't do that. I will never be able to do that again.

A fair comparison starts on the day of my injury—July 6th, 1999. If I compare where I am now to where I started, then wow, what a difference. I have made stunning progress since that date.

When I compare where I am now to where I was five years ago, ten years ago, twenty years ago, or twenty-five years ago, I don't feel small, inferior, or less than. I feel proud, accomplished, confident, and resilient.

Comparison can be used to lift ourselves up, if we do it right.

Comparison didn't just loom large when I thought about my old self. It also showed up when I looked at others on the brain injury journey. Whenever I heard about someone who had returned to work, I wondered, *What's wrong with me?*, *Why can't I do that?* and *Am I not trying hard enough?*

Just like it's not fair to compare our pre and post injury selves, it's also not fair to compare our brain injuries to others' brain injuries. Everyone's injury is unique, and everyone's path is unique.

When that comparison thief creeps into my thoughts, I remind myself that all I can focus on is my own journey, at my own pace.

With that said, when done fairly, comparing ourselves to others' brain injuries can provide inspiration. For example, I got over my denial about needing to use strategies because I was inspired by how another survivor used them to make her life better. I was inspired to become a speaker and author because of the example of my mentor.

When I think about the example those two brain injury survivors set for me, I don't feel small or inferior to them. I feel grateful they lit a path for me. I now feel called to use my experience to light a path for others the way they did for me.

Comparison can be a tool for inspiration, if we choose to use it that way.

As I've become involved on brain injury committees that include professionals, I've discovered that other women my age trigger my comparison thief. When I see all they've accomplished over the long careers they've built, I feel envy and grief for the experience I missed out on. I wonder what my career might have been. I was 32 at the time of my brain injury. My career ended almost before it began.

One would think that reflecting on my post-brain injury accomplishments would tame this comparison thief. After all, I am proud of what I've achieved. However, that doesn't help me feel better in this circumstance.

What does help is to talk to other long-term brain injury survivors, especially those who lost their careers early. Receiving empathy from those who understand helps me know I am not alone in how I feel. I find strength in being part of a community. Through that sense of community, the pain of that comparison is fading.

Comparison can strengthen us, when it's supported by community and compassion.

Comparison doesn't have to be a thief. We can use it to lift ourselves up, to inspire us, and to strengthen us.

Making It Your Own: Applying Silver Learnings

Take a few moments to think about how comparison has influenced your brain injury journey. The questions and action item below are designed to help you connect your experience to the key ideas from this lesson: learning to recognize unfair comparisons, finding pride in progress, and finding inspiration in others' stories.

Section 1: Individual Reflection Questions

- When do I notice myself making comparisons the most?

- What comparisons make me feel discouraged or small?

- What comparisons help me feel proud or inspired?

Section 2: Group Discussion Questions

- What do you say to yourself when you start making unfair comparisons?

- What helps you remember how far you've come?

00000000000

- Has hearing someone else's brain injury story ever helped you feel better about your own journey?

Section 3: Action Item—Suggestion for a Next Step after Reading Lesson 10

- Identify an Inspiration Role Model

  o Think of someone whose story or journey inspires you, such as another brain injury survivor, a mentor, family member, or friend.

  o Take one small step to share how this person has lit a path for you. For example:
    - Send them a brief message (phone, email, text, social media)
    - Mention them in a support group or family discussion
    - Say their name out loud to yourself and acknowledge their influence

105

11.

Even with Strategies,
Expect Your Brain to be Inconsistent

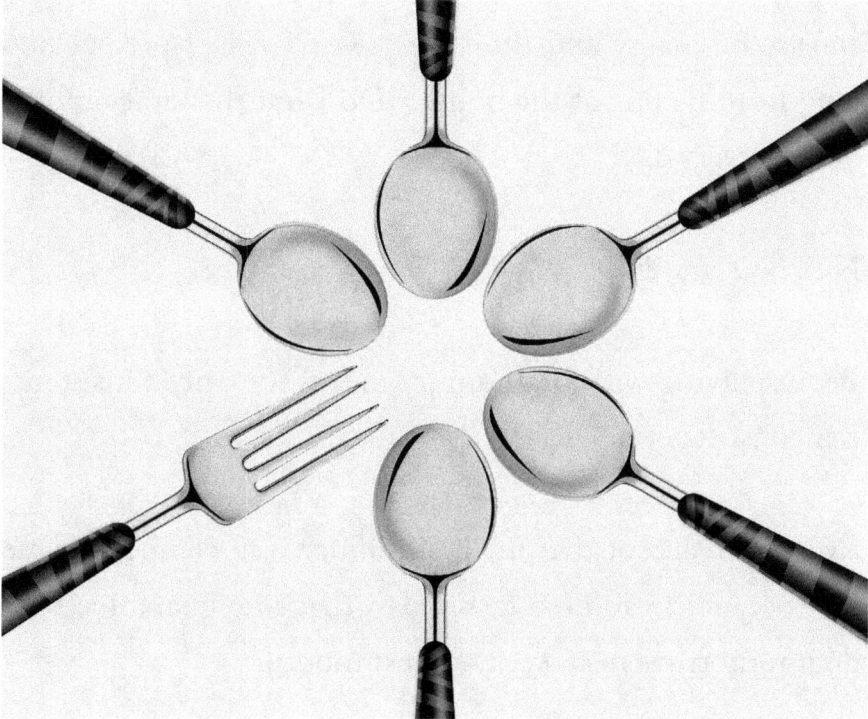

Am I embracing strategies? Yes, I use numerous strategies every day.

Am I pacing myself? Yes, I am careful not to schedule too many activities too close together.

Am I reading my brain injury's signs for overload? Yes, I know how to pay attention to the signals my brain gives that I need to stop and rest.

Because I've learned how to live with my injury over the last twenty-five years, does my brain then reward me with consistent energy and thinking power? Can I predict how long I can be out of the house? Do I rest the same amount of time every day?

NO, NO, and NO!

Because living with brain injury means the only consistency is inconsistency.

I've had to accept that my brain injury is in charge, not me. Just because I can do a task today, that's no guarantee I can do it tomorrow, next week, or next month.

When my brain injury says it's time to stop an activity, I am done. It doesn't matter what I want to do, need to do, or planned to do. It doesn't matter where I am, who I'm with, or how much I want to continue.

Accepting my brain's inconsistency was difficult for me. As a Type A personality, I struggled with feeling like I'd lost control of my life. One of my definitions of being an adult and a professional was getting the job done no matter what, with a high level of consistency and quality. After my brain injury, I could no longer meet that standard.

To cope with this hard truth, I've had to change my expectations. I've learned to go with the flow more, to let my brain set the pace, and to be okay when I'm spending time resting on the couch.

While learning to accept inconsistency has been important, life's demands don't stop. There are still deadlines to meet, appointments to keep, and commitments to honor. How can we balance an unpredictable brain with the realities of everyday life?

One of my strategies is to arrange my schedule so I have the best chance for success. If there are too many deadlines or commitments in a day or week, there is a higher likelihood I'll overload and not be able to meet them.

Generally, I schedule one or two activities a day. I reserve the morning for my most challenging cognitive tasks, since that's when my brain is at its best. At least one day a week, I schedule nothing, to give my brain a chance to recover.

Then, I plan, plan, plan, rest, rest, rest and ask, ask, ask. I repeat those words because these are strategies I use over and over again. Planning, resting and asking support my brain and help reduce the inconsistency I still deal with.

The plan, rest, ask strategy is key to my ability to accomplish big tasks. Because even though we live with brain injury, we all deserve the chance to do something big, whatever that may mean for us.

Creating *Silver Learnings* is an example of something big for me. It began as a conference speech before I turned it into this book.

Preparing *Silver Learnings* as a speech was a task that came with a deadline, was an appointment to keep, and an important commitment to honor. Here's how the plan, rest, ask strategies helped me accomplish it.

Strategy 1—Plan with plenty of time.

When a task is extra important to complete, allotting extra time reduces the chance that inconsistency will get in the way. Overload is more likely when we push too hard and do things last minute.

I knew I wanted to honor my twenty-five-year brain injury anniversary, so I started working on the twenty-five lessons in early 2024, even before I knew they would be a speech.

To do that, I scheduled writing mornings twice a week. Could I always write twice a week? No, because my brain is inconsistent. But because I had plenty of time, the inconsistency didn't matter as much.

Strategy 2—Allow extra rest time.

When a task is especially important to complete, it's likely especially exhausting too. Building in time for additional brain rest is just as important as planning ahead, making it more likely our brains will stay consistent.

Of the three strategies, I struggle with this one the most. Once I found out *Silver Learnings* would be a speech, I jumped into extra cognitive work without scheduling extra rest. That led to overload and a couple weeks off to recover. But because I still had enough time, that was okay.

Strategy 3—Ask for help.

When tasks exceed what our brains can do, there's a higher risk of overload and inconsistency. Help from others enables us to better manage the cognitive load and increases our capacity.

Preparing my *Silver Learnings* speech was a big endeavor. It was a talk with many parts weaving together. There were twenty-five lessons to write, accompanying graphics to find, a video to create, and live polling to learn. It was a presentation unlike any I'd done before.

There were numerous times throughout the process when I got overwhelmed and overloaded. My team of friends, family, and professionals told me when I was doing too much and needed to rest more. They offered meals. They listened and talked me through the steps to put the speech together, offered encouragement, gave feedback on drafts, and listened to me practice. Their many forms of assistance not only made the speech better; they also supported me and my brain injury.

The plan/rest/ask strategies worked. I did give the speech, and it was a success, even with a brain that was inconsistent!

The reality that our brains are inconsistent, even with strategies, is a hard truth that brain injury survivors face. The more we can accept and adapt to the unpredictable rhythm that is life with brain injury, the more we can find peace, resilience, and new ways to thrive.

Making It Your Own: Applying Silver Learnings

This space invites you to explore your thoughts and feelings about coping with brain inconsistency. The questions and action item below are designed to help you connect your experience to the key ideas from this lesson: accepting unpredictability, adjusting expectations, adapting with strategies, and honoring limits.

Section 1: Individual Reflection Questions

- How do I feel when I can't count on my brain to do what I've planned?

- What expectation might I need to change in order to accept my brain's inconsistency?

- What is one strategy I could use to help me on bad brain days?

Section 2: Group Discussion Questions

- What do you wish others understood about brain injury inconsistency?

- What can you do to prepare for your brain's inconsistency?

- How do you bounce back after a bad brain day? What helps you recover?

Section 3: Action Item—Suggestion for a Next Step after Reading Lesson 11

- Support your Brain

  o Pick one activity where your brain's inconsistency causes you stress. It could be something from your daily routine or a big, one-time project.

  o Use these strategies to support your brain:
    - *Plan*: Build in as much flexibility as possible. Give yourself more time than you think you'll need.
    - *Rest*: Schedule extra downtime before and/or after the task.
    - *Ask*: Decide who you could ask for support and what kind of help would make the most difference.

SECTION THREE:

HELPFUL MINDSETS

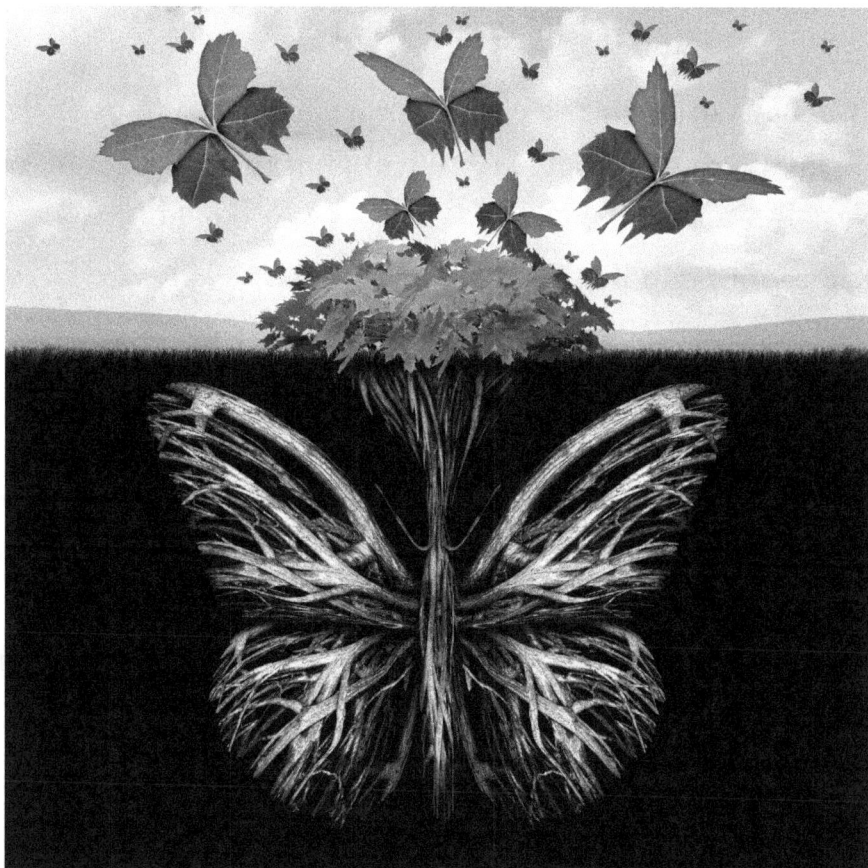

Lightspring/Shutterstock.com

How we think about our situation matters. Our thoughts—our mindsets—are like the roots of a tree, invisible below the surface, but still shaping the structure of our lives. Just as roots anchor a tree, mindsets anchor our beliefs, decisions, and actions.

Our mindsets have power. Just as strong roots nourish a tree and allow it to stand tall and weather storms, helpful mindsets strengthen us and increase our resilience.

We may not be able to change what's happened to us or the brain injury symptoms we live with, but that does not mean we are powerless. We <u>can</u> change our thoughts. We <u>can</u> choose our mindsets.

When my life was uprooted after brain injury, I had to begin anew. The mindsets that had guided me before my injury no longer applied. I had to put down new roots. Below are four mindsets that anchor my new life after brain injury:

- There is no correct path: Each person's journey will be unique
- Where you are today is not where you will always be: Change is slow, but possible
- It's not about getting back to who you were: Focus on who you are now
- A life changed does not mean a life ruined

Just as it takes time for tree roots to establish, so too it takes time for new mindsets to take root. Gradually, these mindsets can help us grow into our new lives as brain injury survivors.

Mindsets are the roots that give us the strength to soar.

12.

There is No Correct Path:
Each Person's Journey will be Unique

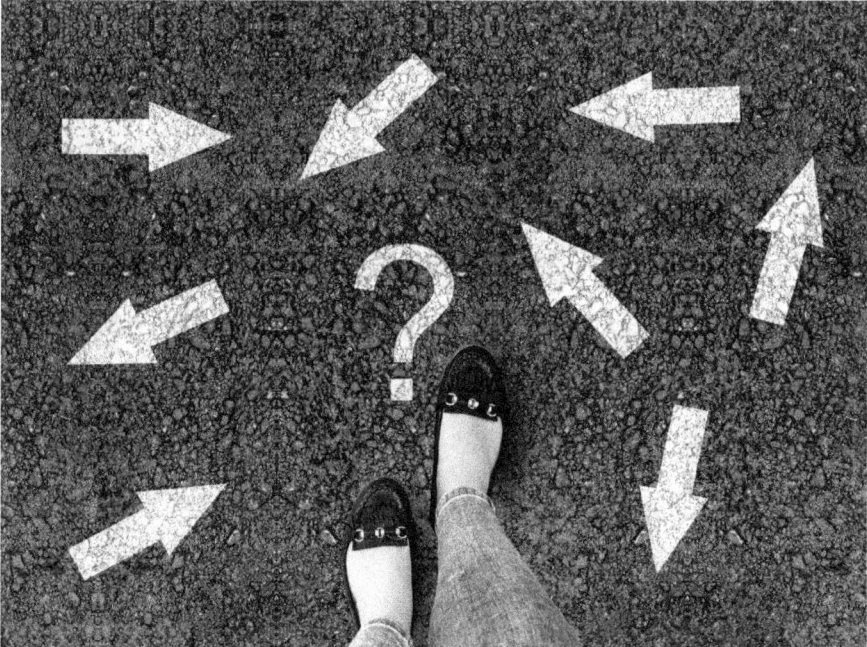

GagoDesign/Shutterstock.com

After an event that impacts us as profoundly as brain injury does, it's natural to look for and to want some sense of certainty. We want a definitive direction to follow. We want a way out of the darkness. We want a way back to our old lives and our old selves.

121

In the early months and years after my brain injury, I desperately wanted someone to provide me with a step-by-step plan. I assumed brain injury would follow a predictable course similar to other injuries and illnesses, with a set treatment plan, a recovery timeline, and a clear path back to normal.

Instead of that clear path, I found a boulder-strewn road full of dead ends, frustrating setbacks, and an uncertain future. While I found helpful treatments and made some progress, the process was haphazard. I often worried I was holding back my recovery because I hadn't discovered the *correct* sequence of therapies. I was frustrated because no one could give me the answers I needed.

What I wanted was something no one could give me—a clearly marked, correct path. The certainty I craved just isn't part of this journey.

There is a lot of ambiguity in brain injury. Every brain is different. Every injury is different. There is no single timeline, standard route, or guaranteed treatment. What works for one person might not work for another. No one knows how much we will recover. Hard work and therapies can help, but they don't promise a return to our old lives and selves. Many of us end up with some permanent challenges. Which exact challenges? How severe? Unknown.

Many of us, me included, struggle with all those unknowns. We need something tangible to hold on to.

This lesson's mindset provides that something tangible, a buffer against brain injury's uncertainties. There may not be a correct path through brain injury, but we can take comfort in knowing there is *a* path for each of us.

Once we let go of searching for that mythical correct path, we can focus on finding our own unique path.

Although our individual paths through brain injury will be different, I think there are some common truths to hold on to. These truths are markers that can anchor and guide us as we navigate our own way forward.

Here are some of the truths I've learned in my journey:

- *It will take time*: There are many brain injury treatment options out there, but often it takes a long time to find them. Progress happens slowly. Patience and persistence are required.

- *Trial and error is part of the process*: Some treatments and strategies will help; some won't. Often there's no way to know until we try. A willingness to experiment—with guidance as needed—and to learn along the way can help move us forward.

- *Progress doesn't move in a straight line*: Ups and downs are normal. Some days we move forward; other days we slide back. Setbacks don't mean failure; they are just part of the brain injury path.

- *It's never too late to try something new*: Even years after injury, new strategies or approaches can make a difference. Timing matters, and what didn't help before might be helpful now.

- *The brain can keep healing*: Neuroplasticity is real; our brains can change, grow, and adapt. We may never be the same as we were, but even small amounts of progress can lead to meaningful improvements in daily life.

Holding on to these truths helps me to better accept all the unknowns that come with brain injury.

Letting go of searching for certainty and embracing ambiguity is part of the brain injury journey. This mindset can help us do that.

Making It Your Own: Applying Silver Learnings

This section encourages you to reflect on your brain injury path. The questions and action item below are designed to help you connect your experience to the key ideas from this lesson: wanting certainty, coping with ambiguity, and learning to embrace one's unique journey.

Section 1: Individual Reflection Questions

- Have I been hoping for the certainty of a *right* way to recover from brain injury?

- What feelings come up when I acknowledge there is no one-size-fits-all path for brain injury?

- What helps me move forward, even if I'm unsure where I'm headed?

Section 2: Group Discussion Questions

- What helps you let go of searching for a certain path through brain injury?

- Has there been a time when your path changed in a way you didn't expect?

- What is one belief or mindset that keeps you moving forward?

Section 3: Action Item—Suggestion for a Next Step after Reading Lesson 12

- Many Ways Forward

  o Choose one small action from the list below. Each is a metaphorical reminder that there are many paths.
    - Walk or drive a different route than usual
    - Watch the clouds move across the sky
    - Sit in a different chair than usual
    - Observe how a squirrel moves for a few minutes
    - Move one item in your home to a new spot
    - Switch up the order of your usual routine
    - Watch something float through the air, like a bubble, leaf, or balloon

13.

Where You Are Today
Is Not Where You Will Always Be:
Change is Slow, But Possible

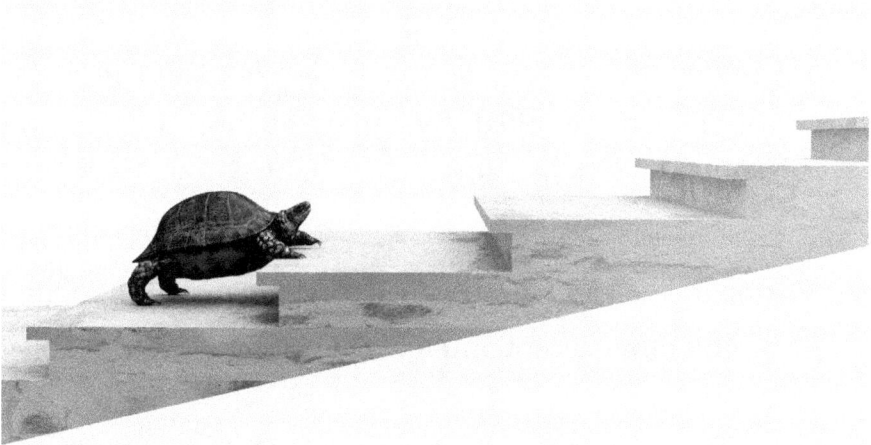

denisgo/Shutterstock.com

Here is a snapshot of what a few pieces of life were like for me in the first few years after my brain injury:

1. I napped four times a day.

2. I had a constant headache.

3. My morning shower exhausted me so much I had to take a nap afterwards.

4. I ate cottage cheese for dinner many nights because shopping for food, planning what to make, and then cooking a meal was too difficult.

5. The noise from planes going over my house seemed so loud that I would duck, scream, and sometimes fall from the sound, even when I was inside.

6. Family and friends had to rescue me from places so often that we joked my car spent more nights away from home than I did.

7. I felt like brain injury had broken me; I thought I could never accept and like the new me.

8. I struggled to give a 5-minute talk about my brain injury experience during a workshop at the Maine Brain Injury Conference.

9. I wrote a few poems about my brain injury.

Here is where I am today regarding those same pieces of life:

1. I still nap every day, but now it's usually once a day. Sometimes I rest twice a day and sometimes I'm on the couch all afternoon.

2. I no longer have headaches.

3. Morning showers don't exhaust me.

4. I have strategies for shopping, meal planning, and cooking. Cottage cheese is mostly a breakfast item, although it does sneak back in for dinner on bad brain days, when my symptoms are worse.

5. I am still sound sensitive and need to use earplugs when out in the world, but my tolerance has improved. Inside or outside, overhead plane noises don't bother me.

6. Family and friends do still rescue me, but that happens more occasionally now. I am better at managing my brain injury.

7. Brain injury did not break me; it made me stronger. I did come to terms with it and learned to like the new me.

8. I now give hour-long speeches and have keynoted in multiple states.

9. I have written two books about brain injury. A line from one of my early poems ended up being the title of my first book, *To Root & To Rise: Accepting Brain Injury*.

I still have a brain injury, but where I was before is not where I am now.

In those early years, as back-to-normal slips away, frustration and grief can outweigh hope. When we are in the midst of all that awfulness, it can feel like life will always be this bad. This lesson's mindset reminds us that is not true. Life is always changing.

When life is challenging, it is important to believe it can get better, even if in the moment we can't see how that will happen. Believing in the possibility of a brighter future can help us through the dark times.

With that said, there is a tortoise in the picture that opens this lesson for a reason. The pace of brain injury progress can be excruciatingly, frustratingly slow. It has taken me twenty-five years to improve to this point.

We can't control the pace of progress. I learned long ago that setting deadlines for improvement does not work, especially for brain injury.

Change happens on its own slow timeline. But slow is still movement. Slow is still progress.

It's important to note the tortoise in the picture is in the process of climbing; it is moving. Change doesn't occur by sitting back and waiting for it to happen. We have to work for every bit of progress we make in order to see change in our lives.

On the bad days, when all we can see is the heartbreak in front of us, this mindset helps us to keep things in perspective, to remember the long view, and to keep slowly climbing upward.

Making It Your Own: Applying Silver Learnings

Here's an opportunity to think about the slow pace of progress after brain injury. The questions and action item below are designed to help you connect your experience to the key ideas from this lesson: progress is possible, small steps add up, and change takes effort.

Section 1: Individual Reflection Questions

- When my brain injury was new, what did I think progress would look like?

- What is one thing I can do now that I couldn't do early in my brain injury journey?

- What is one thing I've accomplished since my brain injury because I kept working at it?

Section 2: Group Discussion Questions

- Why do you think it's hard to notice slow progress?

- What helps you hold on to hope when progress is slow or doesn't seem to be happening?

- What is something that has changed for the better since your brain injury?

Section 3: Action Item—Suggestion for a Next Step after Reading Lesson 13

- Acknowledge an Accomplishment

  o Think of one thing you can do now that you couldn't do early in your brain injury journey.

  o Choose a way to recognize that accomplishment. For example:
    - Take a photo
    - Make a video
    - Write a short note
    - Post on social media
    - Tell someone

14.

It's Not About Getting Back to Who You Were: Focus on Who You Are Now

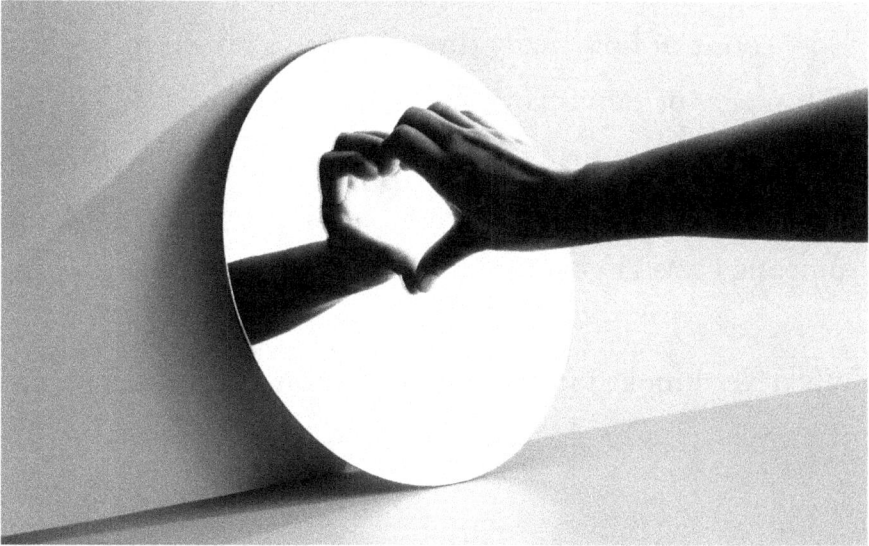

Many of us may dislike or even hate the new people brain injury turns us into. How can we learn to like our new selves? The process begins with this two-part mindset.

It's not about getting back to who you were is about letting go of the past. *Focus on who you are now* is about choosing to live in the present. Neither one is easy to do, but both are essential.

For me, the shift from a focus on the past to a focus on the present took time, help, and many stumbles. Letting go of the past meant working through denial first, especially the belief that if I just tried hard enough, I could return to who I was.

I lost count of how many times I tried to return to teaching and music, of how many situations I tried to fake my way through, of how many times I pretended I was old Carole who didn't have a brain injury. The more I tried to be someone I wasn't anymore, the more my life fell apart.

Whenever I looked in the mirror, I felt like a cracked version of myself—flawed, damaged, and despised.

When we try to be who we're not anymore, we often end up disappointed, discouraged, and feeling less than.

It is a huge switch to go from trying to get back to who we were, to focusing on who we are now. But in that switch is also where we can find the power to like who we see in the mirror and the power to create new lives, as we are.

That transition from past to present can be scary too, especially at first. As we realize that brain injury has changed us and we're not going back to who we were, we may wonder, *If I am not who I was before, then who am I now?*

That was one of my challenges. I knew who I was before my car accident, but brain injury made me a stranger to myself. I needed solid ground to stand on while I slowly found my footing as the new me.

One strategy that helped me over time was writing a series of *Who am I now?* statements. These were words I could live by, even when I didn't know who I was anymore. They served as a temporary self while I was gradually building my new identity and finding my path forward.

Here are a few of my *Who am I now?* statements:

- *I honor my mental fatigue and structure my activities accordingly.*
- *I find what brings me joy and meaning.*
- *Anytime can be nap time, and that's okay.*
- *I celebrate my successes, no matter how small.*

These statements gave me a new self to focus on, a Carole anchored in the present. As this new self slowly emerged, I stopped seeing the cracked version of my old self in the mirror. Instead, I saw a new, whole self—one I could like, one who could gradually create a new life for herself.

That's the power of this mindset. It is only when we turn away from the past and focus on the present that we have any hope of creating a new future.

Making It Your Own: Applying Silver Learnings

This section invites you to reflect on letting go of the past and living in the present. The questions and action item below are designed to help you connect your experience to the key ideas from this lesson: facing the challenges that come with brain injury, learning to value one's new self, and adapting to a changed present.

Section 1: Individual Reflection Questions

- How do I feel when I think about who I was before my brain injury?

- What makes it hard to move on from the old me?

- What do I like or value about the person I am now?

Section 2: Group Discussion Questions

- Which statement fits you best right now: I hate the new me, I like new me, or I'm somewhere in the middle?

- What helps you stay focused on the present and who you are now?

- What is something new about yourself that you are proud of?

Section 3: Action Item—Suggestion for a Next Step after Reading Lesson 14

- Create Your Own *Who am I now?* Statements

  o Jot down 2-3 simple statements that are true about you right now. Here are a few examples to get your thinking started:
    - *I need more rest now and I'm learning to honor that*
    - *I take things one step at a time, and that's okay*
    - *I am more patient because of what I've been through*
    - *I can still help others, just in different ways*
    - *I ask for help when I need it*

  o Keep these statements somewhere easily visible— on your phone, fridge, or desk—to remind yourself of the person you are now.

15.

A Life Changed Does Not Mean a Life Ruined

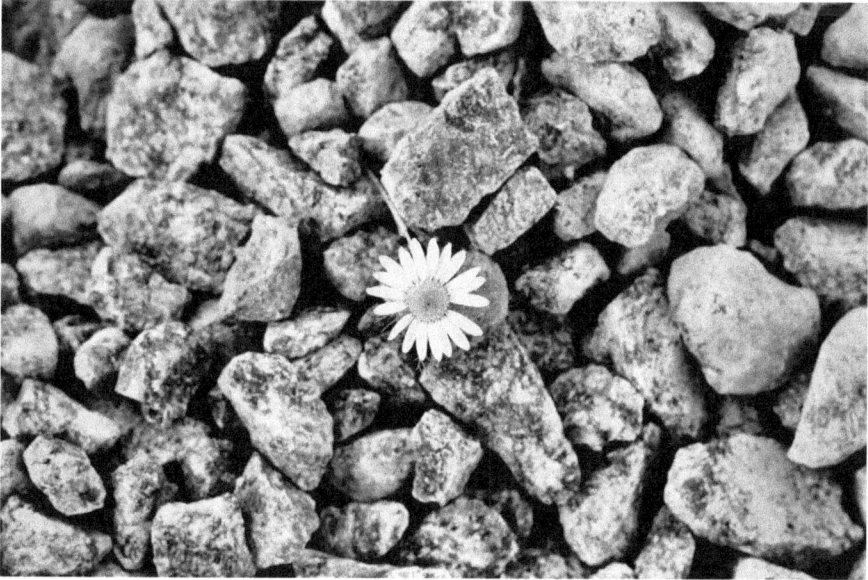

Brain injury is a wrecking ball that smashes through our lives. It demolishes who we are, who we thought we were going to be, the plans we'd made, and the future we'd hoped for.

That is a lot of rubble to cope with. We get to stand in the shattered pieces of what was and what will never be. We get to be in shock, to feel angry, overwhelmed, and scared. We get to grieve everything we've lost.

141

Many of us have wondered, *Is my life ruined now?* It was a thought I had, while I contemplated the rubble of my own changed life, unsure what to do.

When we're surrounded by the wreckage of our lives and selves, it can be hard to see a way out. There's a real danger of getting trapped in the anger, sadness, grief, and longing for what was.

We need a light to hold on to. This mindset can give us one glimmer of hope.

A life changed is <u>not</u> a life ruined. A life changed is simply a life changed. It's important to believe new growth can emerge from the rubble.

We can rebuild our lives. It will take time, it will be hard work, and there will be setbacks.

The new life we create after brain injury will be different than our old life. There is no way for it to be the same. Brain injury changes us.

One thing I've learned is that different doesn't have to mean bad, less than, or ruined. Different is just different.

If we judge our new lives by the standards of our old ones, they will always come up short; they will always seem ruined.

Our new lives need to grow and build, in their own way, and in their own time.

Rubble can be repurposed and used as building blocks to create something new. This is true in our lives too. For example, I was a teacher in my old life. Brain injury destroyed my ability to teach the way I used to. However, I've been able to take that debris and make something new. I am a teacher again, but in a different way. The way I taught before was valuable and the way I teach now is valuable.

My life is changed, but it is not ruined.

This mindset reminds us that the words we use matter and how we look at our situation matters.

If we stay stuck in the rubble, believing our life is ruined, it will become a self-fulfilling prophecy and yes, life will be ruined.

We don't need to have all the steps figured out. We don't need an exact blueprint for how to rebuild our lives. What we do need is a solid foundation—the belief that it is possible.

That belief can make the difference between a life ruined and a life rebuilt.

Making It Your Own: Applying Silver Learnings

Take a moment to reflect how your life has changed since brain injury. The questions and action item below are designed to help you connect your experience to the key ideas from this lesson: acknowledging loss, shifting perspective, and finding hope in what is still possible.

Section 1: Individual Reflection Questions

- What word describes how I see my life after brain injury—ruined, changed, or something else?

- What parts of my life changed the most after my brain injury?

- What helps me believe my life is not ruined?

Section 2: Group Discussion Questions

- How have you grown since your brain injury?

- How are you rebuilding your life?

- Have you been able to use any parts of your old life in a different way? How so?

Section 3: Action Item—Suggestion for a Next Step after Reading Lesson 15

- Take One Rebuilding Step

  o Choose an activity you've been putting off. For example:
    - A phone call, text, email, or appointment
    - A task at home
    - Asking someone for help
    - Going to a new place
    - Attending a virtual event
    - Trying something fun
    - Learning a new skill

  o Break the activity down into one small step you can take today (If needed, ask for help with this).

  o Take the step.

  o Acknowledge out loud that you are rebuilding your life, one step at a time.

SECTION FOUR:

ACCEPTING A NEW SELF

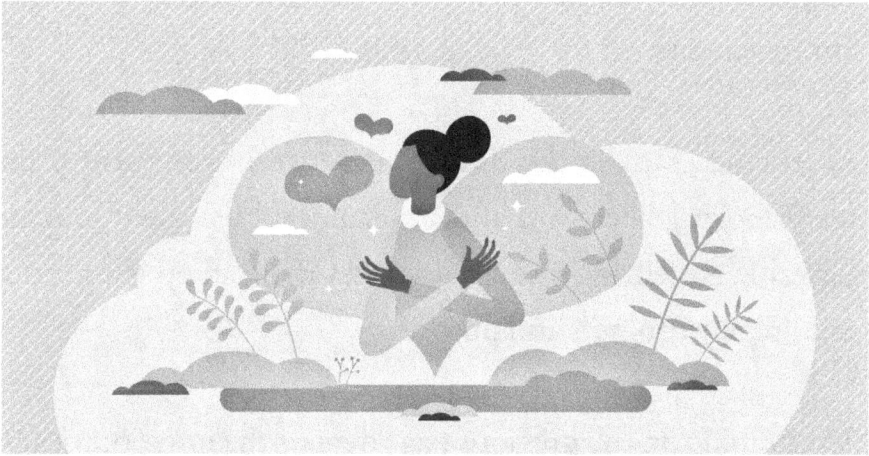

Brain injury slices our lives in two. It is the marker that divides old life from new life, old self from new self. The difference is often dramatic and profound.

Coming to terms with a new self is a key piece of the brain injury journey. It is also one of the most challenging pieces. Coming to self-acceptance is a gradual process that takes years for many of us.

Accepting a new self doesn't mean we have to like what's happened to us. We can accept who we are now and wish that brain injury had never happened, both at the same time.

Coming to terms with brain injury doesn't mean the end of progress. We can accept a new self and continue making improvements.

Acceptance can be the difference between a mournful life spent looking backward and a meaningful life spent looking forward. Accepting a new self is a key that can open the door to a life of happiness and purpose.

The graphic on the previous page depicts the inner peace and serenity that can come with accepting ourselves as we are.

Here are four lessons that helped me gradually learn to accept my new self after brain injury:

- Look at all experience as a teacher
- What <u>can</u> you do? Find something the new you is good at
- Start small, find success and build on it
- Connect with others who share the journey

Accepting our new selves may not change our brain injury symptoms, but it can change how we experience those symptoms and how we think about ourselves.

16.

Look at All Experience as a Teacher

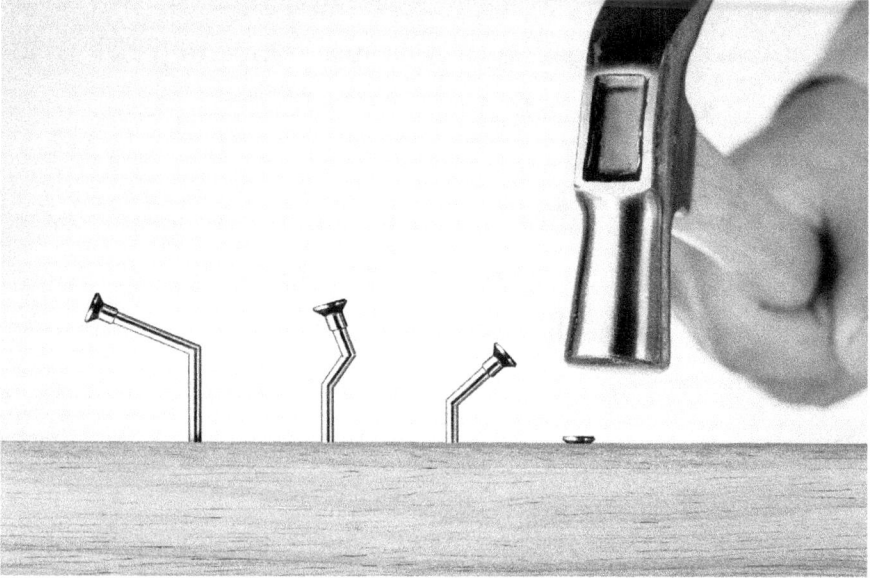

Coming to terms with brain injury and accepting our new selves is a process that can take years for many of us. After my brain injury, I felt stuck for a long time, lost in what felt like a never-ending grief over the end of my old life. I was unsure how to move forward as the new me and uncertain what my future was going to bring.

There were many, many times when I thought I was not capable of coming to terms with brain injury. My journal was full of statements such as, *I do not accept this, I hate the person I am now,* and *I am not strong enough for this.*

But even while all that doubt was going on, I <u>was</u> slowly coming to terms with my new life and my new self. Acceptance was growing; it was just happening below my conscious awareness at first.

What I was conscious of was learning. At a time when embracing who I had become felt impossible, one thing I could whole-heartedly embrace was this lesson—*Look at all experience as a teacher.* And that made a huge difference in my journey.

My experience in school had been that I learned the most from my toughest teachers—the ones who challenged me, and the ones who recognized that learning can happen in the midst of struggle.

I believed this translated to life beyond school. Our toughest, most challenging experiences can provide rich, meaningful opportunities for learning.

The picture opening this chapter echoes that idea. Each crooked nail reflects a struggle and a lesson learned from it.

Brain injury gave me more than my share of crooked nail moments. It was by far my toughest, most challenging teacher ever. But I was okay with that idea, because learning was a process I trusted.

In times of uncertainty, we need something to hold on to. Looking at my brain injury experience as a teacher—that was something I <u>could</u> do, something I could grasp on to.

What I learned from brain injury ultimately played a role in gradually helping me to accept it.

These journal entries from my early years after brain injury show what I was learning in real time:

I'm learning I need to change what I'm working toward. I've been thinking that until and unless I can get back to my pre-injury abilities, I'm damaged goods. I judge myself by how close I'm getting to my pre-injury status. That's an impossible standard to achieve. I am forever changed.

I'm realizing that moving on doesn't mean the sadness and loss completely go away. They just become a smaller segment of my daily existence. For a long time, I've judged myself harshly whenever those feelings came up. I'm gradually learning that

153

victory doesn't come from not having those feelings, but rather from knowing how to deal with them.

I feel vulnerable, like my daffodils in the garden, bent low by the press of the rain. My daffodils may be bent over, but they have lost none of their brightness. I'm learning the same is true of me. I am bent but not broken. My life is not ruined, just changed. It will only be ruined if I allow myself to look at it that way.

I'm learning that the progress I continue to make isn't about regaining the old Carole. It's about creating the new Carole.

When I wrote those journal entries, I had no idea how to accept my new self. However, I think it's clear from my writing that as I was learning and looking at brain injury as a teacher, I was also gradually moving toward self-acceptance, one crooked nail at a time.

We may not be ready to accept all the ways brain injury has changed us, but we can choose to learn through the experience. And in time, that learning might lead us somewhere we never thought we could go—toward acceptance.

Making It Your Own: Applying Silver Learnings

Take a few moments to think about how learning from experience—even painful experience like brain injury—can help you move forward. The questions and action item below are designed to help you connect your experience to the key ideas from this lesson: seeing life as a teacher, finding growth in hard times, and moving slowly toward self-acceptance.

Section 1: Individual Reflection Questions

- What is one thing I've learned from brain injury that surprised me?

- Do I think of myself as someone who is still learning and growing?

- What is one way I've grown that I can see now, but didn't recognize at the time?

Section 2: Group Discussion Questions

- Do you think life experience is a good teacher? Why or why not?

- Can you share one brain injury challenge that taught you something meaningful?

- How can listening to each other's stories help us move toward acceptance?

Section 3: Action Item—Suggestion for a Next Step after Reading Lesson 16

- Identify a *Tough Teacher* Lesson

  o Think of one challenge you've faced since your brain injury.

  o Ask yourself:
    - What did I learn from this experience?
    - Did it help me understand myself better?
    - Did it show me something I needed to do differently?

  o There are no wrong answers. This is a way to notice how you've grown, even during tough times.

17.

What <u>Can</u> You Do?
Find Something the New You is Good At

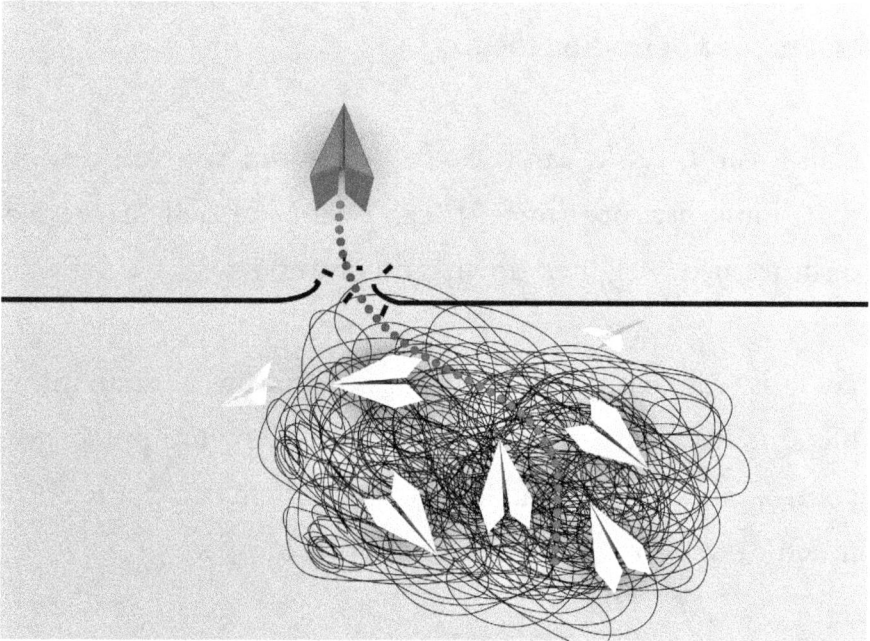

Vector memory/Shutterstock.com

Since my brain injury, I

- Can't work full-time anymore
- Can't be a teacher the way I used to be
- Can't be a musician
- Can't always think clearly or find the words I want to say
- Can't be upright for more than a few hours at a time

- Can't tolerate sound or bright lights
- Can't drive very far or travel long distances on my own

I could list more of my brain injury can'ts, but I think I've included enough to make my point, and I would imagine you're tired of reading them.

Can't, can't, can't, can't, can't. How did you feel reading that long list of things I can't do? I felt depressed, disheartened, weighted down, and powerless.

Yes, it is true that the all-encompassing nature of brain injury fills our lives with numerous can'ts. Many are out of our control, and we are unable to change them, no matter how much we want to. We get to grieve those losses.

As we just experienced, it's easy to get bogged down in all those can'ts. If we live our lives focused mostly on everything we can no longer do, we will stay stuck, like the paper airplanes in the picture on the previous page.

Changing our focus from can't to can is a strategy that can help us break free and rise into a new life. Changing our focus from can't to can helps us to accept our new selves.

Let's try that strategy out and flip the script from can't to can on a couple of my earlier statements.

It is true; I can't work a full-time job. However, I can volunteer to help other survivors. I can serve on brain injury committees. I can make a difference.

It is true; I can't perform as a musician anymore. However, I can now listen to music again. I can now go to concerts again. I can use my background as a musician to influence the flow and rhythm of my writing and speaking.

As you read the can's, how do you feel now? I feel inspired, motivated, and hopeful. That's the power of flipping our focus from can't to can.

When we focus on what we <u>can</u> do, we transform from being powerless and trapped by circumstance to being powerful and action oriented. Self-acceptance grows as we figure out what we're good at now.

Given the magnitude of losses we cope with after brain injury, it's easy to believe we are not good at anything anymore. That was not true for me, and it is not true for you.

Our new selves have talents, ones that may be different from our old selves. I discovered my new self was good at crafts, something I had never done before and had no interest in pre-brain injury.

We may find ourselves using previous skills in new ways after brain injury. I am still a teacher. I still think like an educator. That mindset influences how I write and how I organize my speeches.

I encourage you to make a list of what you <u>can</u> do. Write down as many things as you can think of. It doesn't matter how small or trivial the items on the list may seem. Notice what brings forth an emotion, what sparks your interest, what piques your curiosity. These are clues that can help you find what you're good at now.

As we break free from our can'ts and focus on our can's, we have the chance to rise into our new selves and our new lives.

Making It Your Own: Applying Silver Learnings

This reflection section is about shifting focus from what you can't do to what you can do. The questions and action item below are designed to help you connect your experience to the key ideas from this lesson: acknowledging limitations, identifying abilities, and building a new sense of self.

Section 1: Individual Reflection Questions

- What is something I can't do since my brain injury that has been difficult for me to accept?

- What is something I <u>can</u> do now—either in the same way or a different way?

- Have I discovered any new interests or skills since my brain injury?

Section 2: Group Discussion Questions

- How do you shift your focus from what you can't do to what you can do?

- How has your definition of success changed since your brain injury?

- What qualities or strengths do you value in yourself since your brain injury?

Section 3: Action Item—Suggestion for a Next Step after Reading Lesson 17

- Try a <u>Can</u> Time

  o Pick a morning or afternoon to focus on what you <u>can</u> do.

  o For a few hours (or as long as you're able to), briefly jot down anything, big or small, you are able to do. For example:
    ▪ I made breakfast/lunch
    ▪ I checked my email
    ▪ I called a friend
    ▪ I rested when I needed to

  o Later, reflect on your list.
    ▪ Did anything surprise me?
    ▪ Did I learn anything about myself?

18.

Start Small, Find Success and Build on It

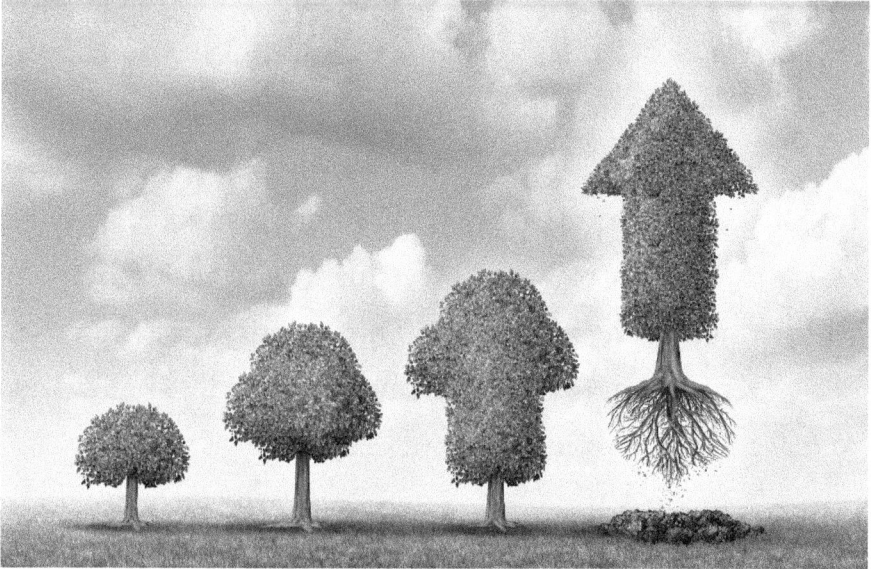

Lightspring/Shutterstock.com

Part of acceptance is coming to terms with a new life after brain injury.

Start Small, Find Success and Build on It, together with Lesson 17 (*What Can You Do?*), form my blueprint for building that new life.

First, we *Start Small*. Small is doable and non-threatening. Small can lead us toward our new lives.

Completing a paint by number of a sun was my first small step toward accepting my new life. A simple craft might not seem life-changing, but it was for me. In fact, I am a speaker and author today because of that paint by number and because of the mantra that is this chapter's lesson: *Start small, find success and build on it.* Small choices we make can gradually lead to unexpected paths.

In 2001, two years after my brain injury, I suddenly wanted to use my hands to create. A small voice inside me kept whispering, *Make something.* This surprised me, because I had never been drawn to crafts before. I didn't know what to make of this new interest, but decided to give it a try.

The paint by number represented the first time I turned away from trying to get back to my old life. Even though I could only work on it for fifteen minutes at a time before needing to rest my brain, it was something I <u>could</u> do. With each stroke of the brush, I was slowly crafting my new life.

I didn't know where that paint by number would lead. I just knew I needed to keep following the whisper and *make something.*

Successfully finishing that first small craft gave me the confidence to try others, including jewelry making, knitting, cross-stitching, and photography. I didn't know it then, but that tiny paint by number would become my first step on a much bigger path.

For each of us, start small will look different. Maybe it's not a whisper, but a quiet pull inside that guides us to *plant something, bake something, write something, paint something, go outdoors, move our body, or connect with someone.* The start small possibilities are as unique as we are.

After brain injury, many of us fail so often that our self-confidence and self-esteem plummet. The more we try—and fail—to return to our old lives, the worse it gets. Repeated failures are not motivating. They are demoralizing.

That's why the second part of this chapter's title is so vital—*Find Success.* Success can be like a shot of adrenaline. Even a small win can spark momentum, remind us what we're capable of, and help us move forward.

Crafts gave me something I hadn't felt since my brain injury—a feeling of accomplishment. With each project, I felt like a success, something I hadn't experienced when I was trying and failing to return to teaching and music.

With crafts, there was no pressure to be who I used to be. There were no comparisons to old Carole, because I was doing something new. There was simply the satisfaction of creating something.

Over time, my small successes with crafts added up. The more I succeeded, the more willing and motivated I was to try small next steps. These included making crafts for family and friends and teaching jewelry making to other brain injury survivors.

Success doesn't just lift our spirits; it can also move us toward new, unexpected lives. Success is the foundation for the third part of my mantra—*Build on It.*

Success with crafts helped me build a new life. Because of the crafts I did, I was invited to participate in a creativity workshop at the Maine Brain Injury Conference in 2003. In addition to displaying my crafts, I also had my first opportunity to speak publicly about my brain injury. My speech was five minutes long, and I was so nervous my knees shook the entire time. But I did it.

Speaking at that conference increased my self-esteem and self-confidence. It showed me the power of using my story to help others and made me feel like there was some value and purpose in all I had been through.

While I was speaking, even though I was nervous, I felt a strong sense of being *home*. For the first time since my car accident in 1999, my way forward was clear. I knew I wanted to do more speaking about brain injury.

It's now been more than two decades since I gave that first five-minute, knee-knocking speech about brain injury. In that time, I've gone from being part of panels, to giving short talks, to organizing workshops, to delivering keynote speeches, to writing two books, to becoming involved in brain injury at the national level.

And it all started with that first paint by number.

Start Small, Find Success and Build on It changed the direction of my life. But this mantra isn't only about big transformations. Sometimes, the small step itself is the victory. Every time we try something new—no matter how small—it is an act of courage. Step by step, that's how we build our lives after brain injury.

Making It Your Own: Applying Silver Learnings

This section encourages you to think about how small steps, success, and growth show up in your life after brain injury. The questions and action item below are designed to help you connect your experience to the key ideas from this lesson: trying something new, recognizing accomplishments, and allowing success to build gradually over time.

Section 1: Individual Reflection Questions

- What is one small thing I've done since my brain injury that I feel proud of?

- What helps me get started when something feels new or difficult?

- What is a success or accomplishment I've had since my brain injury?

Section 2: Group Discussion Questions

- Has a small step ever led you somewhere unexpected?

- What does success look like for you now?

- What helps you keep building on small successes?

Section 3: Action Item—Suggestion for a Next Step after Reading Lesson 18

- Try One New Thing

  o Choose one small, low-pressure activity you haven't tried before. It doesn't need to be creative or involved. Some examples include:
    - Trying a new snack or meal
    - Walking a different route
    - Rearranging one item in your living space
    - Watching a new show or video
    - Saying hello to someone new
    - Trying a different way to relax

  o Notice how trying this small activity makes you feel. Do you want to try more?

  o Give yourself permission to be curious. The goal is to practice starting small.

19.

Connect with Others Who Share the Journey

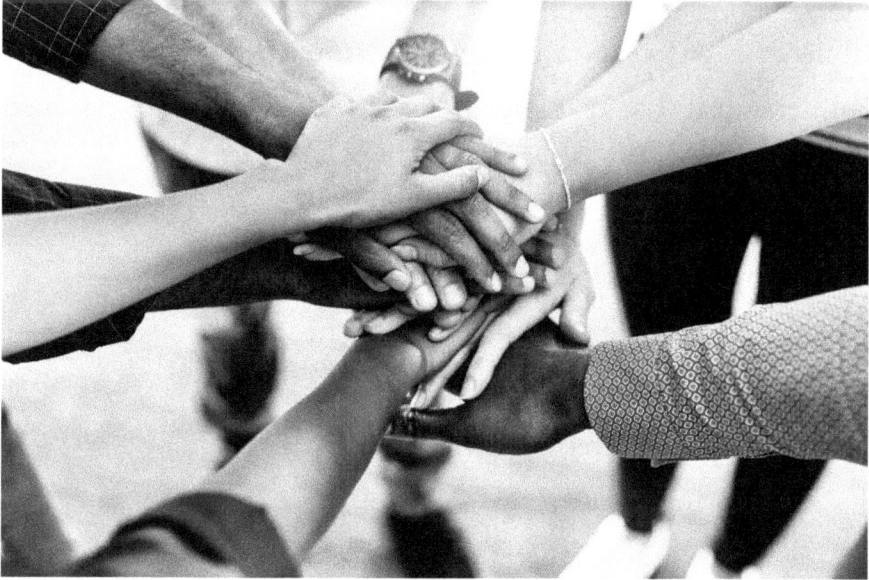

As much as brain injury survivors need our families, friends, and professionals, we also need each other. Our shared experience connects us in a way that sometimes feels almost magical.

There is a special shorthand that happens among brain injury survivors. When I say, *I get tired, I'm overloaded,* or *I forget things,* other survivors hear more than just my words. They also understand the frustration, grief, and challenge packed into those short sentences. They know that although people without brain injuries also get tired, overwhelmed, and forgetful, the experience I am describing is not the same at all.

There is a profound sense of relief when someone understands us at a deep level. It is vital to be seen, recognized, and heard.

Brain injury survivors can help each other by:
- validating each other's experience
- offering camaraderie
- helping each other know that we're not alone
- sharing resources
- modeling strategies

I've experienced all those benefits from connecting with my peers. In the early years after my brain injury, long-term survivors showed me it was possible to accept brain injury, to come to terms with a new self, and to create a fulfilling, different life. Their examples comforted and inspired me.

During times of frustration, sadness, and self-doubt, their stories were a light in the darkness. When I didn't believe in myself, I held on to their examples.

Even now, as a long-term brain injury survivor, it's still important for me to connect with my peers. I cope with daily brain injury symptoms, and sometimes I feel sad and frustrated by what I can't do. Validation from others on the brain injury path makes my journey easier. I don't think we ever outgrow the need for our peers.

There are many ways to connect with others who share our journey. Early on, I was scared to meet other brain injury survivors. I could barely handle my own story and didn't feel ready to cope with listening to other's experiences.

What I could do was slowly read a book by another brain injury survivor. Her words were a safe way for me to begin processing my experience. They began my journey to self-acceptance.

In addition to books, we can listen to podcasts, watch videos by brain injury survivors, and join brain injury groups on social media. These are other non-in-person ways to connect.

There may come a time when we're ready to connect in-person. It takes courage to put ourselves out there and meet our peers.

What worked for me was beginning one-on-one. Once a month, I went to lunch with a friend I met at brain injury rehab. We shared our brain injury stories, challenges, and successes. This was peer support on a scale I could handle at the time.

Then, I began attending a brain injury support group. As part of my rehab program, one of my therapists went with me. She smoothed my way into the group, sat next to me, introduced me to people, and made me feel comfortable. In this group, I found a home as a brain injury survivor. I am now the facilitator of that group.

Over time, other options for connecting with peers in-person can include attending brain injury conferences, getting involved in activities organized by state brain injury associations, advocating for brain injury issues, and joining brain injury boards and committees.

Yes, connecting with others can feel risky. Yes, it can be a vulnerable experience to tell one's story. That's why it's important to connect in ways that match our comfort level.

Stepping back or slowing down can be good strategies to reduce overwhelm and ensure connection happens at a pace that works for us. Not every group or every conversation will be a fit, and that's okay.

Connecting with others is a process, not a one-time event. When we connect in ways that work best for us, based on wherever we are in our journey, the rewards outweigh the risks.

Connection reminds us that we are not alone. In community, we can find understanding, wisdom, and hope. Through that strength, we can begin to accept—and even embrace—our new selves after brain injury.

Making It Your Own: Applying Silver Learnings

This section gives you an opportunity to think about how connecting with other survivors could support your journey. The questions and action item below are designed to help you connect your experience to the key ideas from this lesson: feeling understood, finding ways to connect, and learning from other brain injury survivors.

Section 1: Individual Reflection Questions

- Do I feel nervous about connecting with other brain injury survivors? Why or why not?

- What connection works best for me right now—reading a book, listening to a podcast, watching a video, meeting one-on-one, or joining a group?

- How would connecting with other survivors help me in my brain injury journey?

Section 2: Group Discussion Questions

- How does talking with other brain injury survivors help you feel understood?

- Has hearing another survivor's story ever changed how you see your own journey?

- How could sharing your story help someone else?

Section 3: Action Item—Suggestion for a Next Step after Reading Lesson 19

- Try One Connection Step

  o Choose a form of connection that feels safe and doable for you. For example:
    - Read an article or blog post by a brain injury survivor
    - Watch a survivor's video or listen to a podcast episode
    - Join a brain injury survivor community through social media
    - Attend a virtual or in-person brain injury support group meeting

  o Afterwards, decide if this is something you would do again or if you would like to try another form of connection from the list.

SECTION FIVE:

THRIVING AFTER BRAIN INJURY

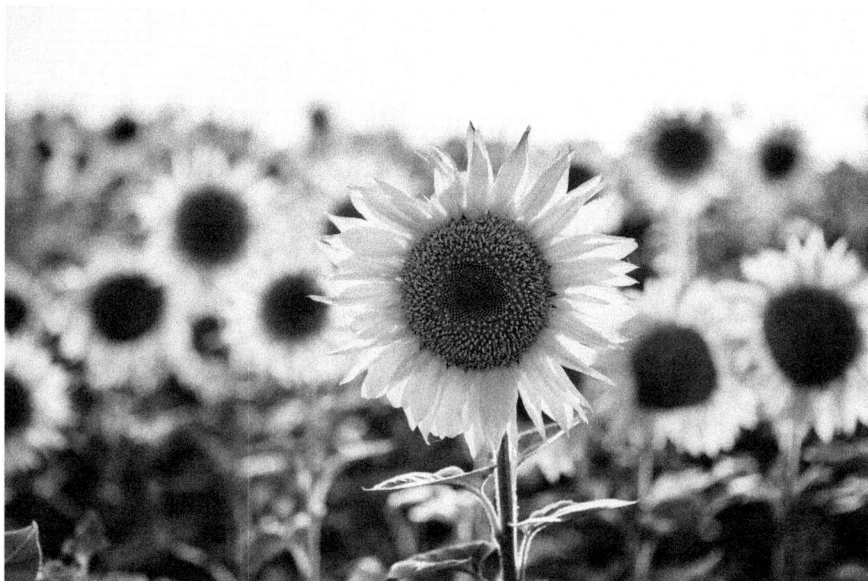

Thriving with brain injury doesn't mean our symptoms disappear or our struggles end. It means we've learned to cope, face hard truths, adopt helpful mindsets, and accept our new selves—all while offering ourselves grace along the way.

Sunflowers are a powerful metaphor for thriving. Even on cloudy days, they turn toward the direction of the sun.

Thriving means orienting ourselves toward the light—toward hope, joy, and growth—even in dark times.

In strong winds and storms, sunflowers bend but do not break. Thriving is believing in our own resilience. Like the sunflower, we can rise and bloom again.

A single sunflower is lovely, but a field of sunflowers is breathtaking. Thriving means finding community, growing alongside others, and drawing strength from connection.

Here are six lessons that have helped me thrive with brain injury:
- Take risks
- Find humor
- Own who you are: Don't apologize for having a disability
- Assemble a team and listen to their advice
- Recognize and celebrate progress
- Make meaning from suffering: Connect to your purpose

Thriving with brain injury isn't about getting everything right all the time. It's about doing our best, learning as we go, trying again, and holding on to hope. It's about turning toward the light and continuing to bloom.

20.

Take Risks

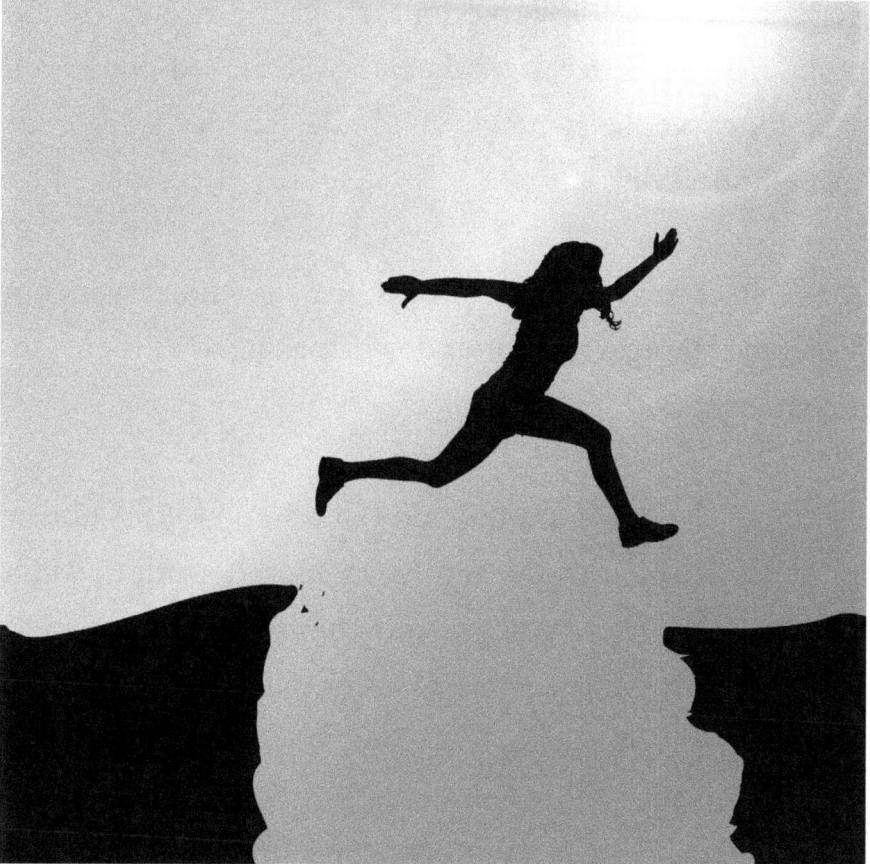

The picture above is dramatic. A woman leaping across a chasm is the very definition of risk taking. But I'm not suggesting anyone take a literal leap like that. It's the symbolism of the leap that matters most. In this chapter, I invite you to focus on the *inner* leap this image represents—

challenging yourself, pushing your boundaries, and expanding your capabilities.

That kind of leap isn't always easy after brain injury. The cognitive, physical, and emotional challenges we live with can make risk taking feel overwhelming. Fear, self-doubt, and hesitation can keep us glued to the familiar side of the metaphorical cliff.

Or maybe you've taken some risks, and they didn't work out. Repeated failures can wear us down, making us cautious, and unwilling to risk again.

All those challenges are real and valid; I don't want to deny or downplay their truth. But here's another truth to add to the mix. We are not going to move forward, and we are not going to thrive unless we step out of our comfort zone and choose to take some risks.

Let me qualify that by adding one key idea: risks with support. Support can transform a risk from something scary into something we can grow from. Support can make thriving possible.

Let me also be very clear about the kind of risks I mean. I'm not talking about reckless or impulsive risks that could jeopardize our health or safety or that of others.

I'm talking about risks that are positive and calculated— challenges that stretch us just enough to build confidence and create new possibilities.

That's why I chose the picture that opens this chapter. The woman is clearly going to make that jump. She's not flinging herself into the unknown with no hope of landing. She's taking a leap she knows she can make—one that will move her forward—not put her in danger.

She is stretching herself just enough to grow.

I took one of those leaps more than two decades ago, when I gave my first five-minute speech at a brain injury conference. It was the first time I publicly shared my story. That leap challenged me, stretched my boundaries, and expanded my capabilities. Because of that leap, I discovered that using my story to help others was a way for me to thrive.

That first speaking experience didn't just boost my confidence; it showed me that growth was possible. With each small step forward, my comfort zone expanded.

As I gradually grew more confident in public speaking, I took on bigger challenges: managing slides, adlibbing, speaking without notes for short talks, encouraging audience participation, and using live polling. Each one felt like a risk, but each one helped me grow.

Planning, practice, strategies, and assistance from others made those risks successful. These kinds of support reduce the chance of failure and increase confidence. They can make the difference between staying stuck and leaping forward. They can also help ensure that when we do leap, we make it to the other side safely and successfully.

Risks can take many forms—physical, mental, emotional, or social. For brain injury survivors, a positive, calculated risk might be trying a new strategy, seeing a different medical provider, getting out of the house, sharing one's story, going to a support group, attending a brain injury conference, attending a social activity, trying a new hobby, or attempting a new exercise.

Risks are individual. What feels risky to one person might feel easy to someone else. What matters is choosing an activity that stretches *you*, that helps *you* grow.

The more supported risks we take, the more our tolerance grows. What once felt impossible could eventually become doable. That first five-minute speech was a big risk for me. It would not be today.

Taking risks can boost our self-confidence and self-esteem, increase our independence, enrich our lives, and help us avoid stagnation. But those benefits only come when we're willing to take the leap.

Thriving after brain injury doesn't happen by staying where it's safe and familiar. Thriving happens through small, supported steps that stretch us. Like the woman leaping from cliff to cliff, we grow stronger and more confident each time we land on new ground. Every leap reminds us that thriving is possible in the life we have now.

Making It Your Own: Applying Silver Learnings

Use this space to think about how risk taking might support your growth after brain injury. The questions and action item below are designed to help you connect your experience to the key ideas from this lesson: exploring one's comfort zone, recognizing boundaries, and building capacity for positive, supported risk.

Section 1: Individual Reflection Questions

- What is one small risk I've taken since my brain injury?

- How did taking that risk feel? Scary, exciting, or something else?

- What support do I need to continue taking positive, calculated risks?

Section 2: Group Discussion Questions

- What is a risk you've taken that helped you grow?

- How do you decide whether a risk is worth taking?

- Has your comfort with taking risks changed since your brain injury? If so, how?

Section 3: Action Item—Suggestion for a Next Step after Reading Lesson 20

- Try a Supported Stretch

  o Choose a small risk you feel ready to take. It should stretch you slightly but not overwhelm you. Examples could include:
    - Trying a new hobby
    - Saying yes to something you usually avoid
    - Sending a message to connect with someone
    - Attending a virtual or in-person brain injury support group
    - Sharing your brain injury story with someone you trust

  o Identify the support you need to help make your risk more likely to succeed. For example:
    - Break the task down into small steps
    - Ask someone to come with you/help you
    - Try the activity when you have enough energy

21.

Find Humor

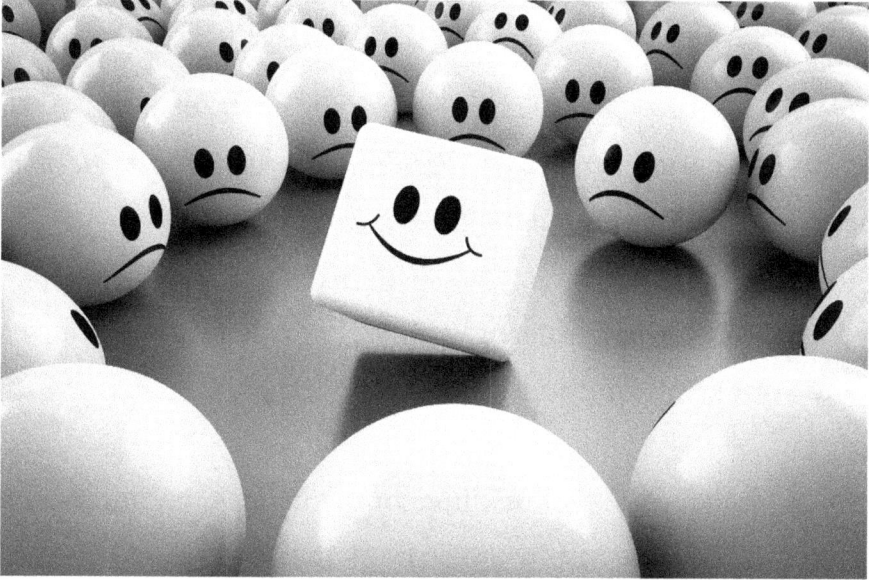

The comedian Charlie Chaplin said, *To truly laugh, you must be able to take your pain and play with it.* In honor of that quote, I'm going to morph into a brain injury comic. Let me try out some of my material on you.

Brain injury memory loss—The gift that keeps on....wait, what?

Memory loss means we can plan our own surprise party...and still be surprised!

Living with brain fog is like trying to stream a movie in low resolution.

Here's a strategy for times when brain fog hits in public. Stare into space with intensity. People will think you're deep in thought instead of lost with no idea what to do!

You might be laughing right now, because you see yourself and your symptoms in these jokes.

Or perhaps you're chuckling, but you feel uncomfortable doing it, because you're not sure if these jokes are mocking brain injury and trivializing the challenges we face.

Or maybe you're outright appalled. After all, brain injury is serious. It changes who we are and rips our lives apart in ways that are anything but funny.

How we react to brain injury humor depends on where we are in our journey, who is using the humor, and the intent behind it. I've learned that firsthand.

When I first met my mentor Bev Bryant about a year after my injury, I was horrified by how she would laugh and joke about her own brain injury. I remember thinking, *Brain injury is* <u>*not*</u> *funny. It is serious, devastating, and life altering.*

Although I couldn't laugh at my brain injury symptoms then, I could see that humor brought joy, creativity, and a sense of strength to Bev and to other long-term survivors I met. Humor helped them thrive.

Just knowing humor was possible stuck with me. It was a light in the darkness, a promise of a way forward.

It took years before I could find that lightness within my own brain injury symptoms. Mark Twain's wisdom applies here: *Humor is tragedy plus time.*

Most of my brain injury humor centers around my most challenging symptom—ongoing, often severe mental fatigue.

When my brain says rest, I must obey, no matter where I am. Sometimes that means resting in public places. Let's just say I've had to get creative with where I lie my head down when fatigue hits.

Here are a few of the many places I've rested:

- On more benches in more coffee shops than I can count
- On floors, when there was no other place to lie down
- In the coffin display room at a funeral home (*Don't worry, I rested on a couch—not in a coffin!*)
- On beds in furniture stores
- On couches in hotel lobbies and bars
- In the middle of a flower garden
- In conference rooms on the House and Senate sides of the U.S. Capitol

Given all that, I tell people I sleep around! My motto is one that Star Trek fans will appreciate—*To boldly nap where no one has napped before!*

Finding humor in a painful situation is a choice. Believe me, when my brain is dragging me down and my only option is to go horizontal in a public space, it's neither fun nor funny. When we choose to find the humorous side of our experience, we claim power over how we tell our story.

We may not be able to control our brain injury symptoms, but we can control how we talk about them. Humor turns the spotlight away from what's damaged and focuses it on resilience.

Finding humor can help us gain perspective. Laughing at our symptoms does not mean we are trivializing them. Instead, laughter allows us to create a healthy distance between us and our challenges, showing that we are not defined solely by our brain injury.

Finding humor can bridge gaps. When we can laugh at our symptoms, it puts us and others at ease. Walls can come down and rapport can increase.

Finding humor can improve health. Research has shown physiological benefits of humor and laughter can include reduced muscle tension, lower blood pressure, reduced pain, increased immunity, reduced stress, and better memory.

Brain injury is still serious, devastating, and life-altering. There will be dark days when humor escapes us. That's okay. Playing with our pain is not about dismissing it. It's about choosing to engage with it differently.

Humor gives us a way to rise above the hard moments, to find connection, and to keep going. It reminds us that even when everything is falling apart, we can still choose to laugh. And in doing that, we do more than survive. We thrive.

Making It Your Own: Applying Silver Learnings

Take a few moments to reflect on the role of humor in your brain injury journey. The questions and action item below are designed to help you connect your experience to the key ideas from this lesson: humor as a tool for resilience, laughter as a source of strength, and the possibility of finding light in dark times.

Section 1: Individual Reflection Questions

- How did I react to the brain injury jokes on pages 189-190? Was I amused, uncomfortable, or appalled?

- Have I ever found humor in my brain injury journey?

- How could humor help me on a hard brain day?

Section 2: Group Discussion Questions

- What are your thoughts about whether it is possible to laugh and still take brain injury seriously?

- Can you think of a time when another survivor's humor helped you feel more understood or less alone?

- How can humor build bridges between people with brain injury and those without?

Section 3: Action Item—Suggestion for a Next Step after Reading Lesson 21

- Give it a Name

  o Think of a frustrating brain injury situation you are ready to *play with*, such as:
    - Forgetting something important
    - Getting overwhelmed in a noisy place
    - Needing to rest in public
    - Saying the wrong word

  o Give that moment a name. For example:
    - A dramatic title: The Great Grocery Store Meltdown
    - A sitcom episode: Season 2, Episode 5: Lost in My Own House
    - A simple phrase: Misfire Monday

  o Naming the moment is a way to *play with the pain*, take away some of its sting, and create a little emotional distance.

22.

Own Who You Are:
Don't Apologize for Having a Disability

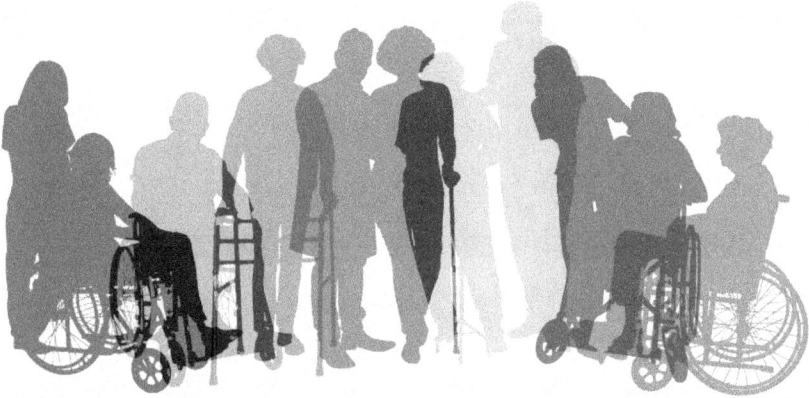

Years ago, at a family gathering, I started to get brain tired. As my symptoms took over—the mental fog, the overwhelm, the confusion—I knew I needed to rest, but I felt awful about leaving.

So, I apologized. Once. Then again, and again.

I felt like I was spoiling the fun. Like my brain injury was an inconvenience and a burden. Like *I* was an inconvenience and a burden.

Later, my sister asked me why I felt the need to apologize so much. Her question caught me off guard, and I didn't have a good answer.

In her gentle way, she reminded me that needing to rest wasn't something to apologize for. It was just what I needed to do.

It was one of those moments when insight arrives all at once. She was right. I had nothing to apologize for. And more than that, I had nothing to be ashamed of.

That day was a turning point. It was time to stop apologizing and start owning who I was.

For many years, I had apologized excessively whenever my brain injury symptoms showed themselves. I apologized when I needed help, when I left events early, or when I couldn't attend at all. I apologized when my emotions spilled over, and I overloaded. I apologized when I needed my earplugs, headphones, sunglasses, or hat. I apologized not just for what I did, but for who I was.

Deep down, I was ashamed of brain injury Carole. Non-disabled Carole was my standard, and because I couldn't live up to who I used to be, I felt the need to apologize—a lot.

Part of thriving is owning who we are—our brain injury symptoms, the accommodations we need, and the strategies we use. We may still struggle. We may still grieve. But we do not need to be ashamed, and we do not need to apologize for living with a disability.

Owning who we are doesn't change our brain injury symptoms, but it can change how we feel about them and how we present ourselves to the world.

Owning who we are says, *Here I am, as I am*, without shame and without embarrassment.

There's an internal power that comes from owning who we are. Here's what that looks like for me now:

- Owning who I am means acknowledging I have brain injury symptoms I can't always control, and sometimes they get the better of me.
- It means knowing I am doing the best I can.
- It means doing what I need to do to take care of myself.
- It means not asking permission for the accommodations I need. If I'm at a gathering and I need to rest, I go rest with no shame attached. I can be sad I'll miss some of it, but there's a difference

between sadness over the circumstance and shame over who I am.

- It means apologizing when I've done something wrong, but not for being who I am now and not for having a disability.

Owning who we are claims our power and gives us strength. It helps us thrive by standing in our truth, just as we are.

Making It Your Own: Applying Silver Learnings

Use this space to explore how shame, apology, and self-perception have influenced your brain injury journey. The questions and action item below are designed to help you connect your experience to the key ideas from this lesson: releasing unnecessary shame, standing in one's truth, and learning to live without apology.

Section 1: Individual Reflection Questions

- How often do I apologize for things related to my brain injury?

- Do I feel like I have to explain or justify my needs?

- What is one thing related to my brain injury I would like to stop apologizing for?

Section 2: Group Discussion Questions

- Why do you think many brain injury survivors feel the need to apologize?

- Has someone ever helped you feel okay about asking for what you need? What happened?

- What does *owning who you are* mean to you in your everyday life?

Section 3: Action Item—Suggestion for a Next Step after Reading Lesson 22

- Try One Unapologetic Act

  o Choose one small thing you usually apologize for—resting, needing help, wearing sunglasses indoors, leaving early—and practice doing it <u>without</u> an apology.

  o Notice how it feels not to apologize. Was it uncomfortable? Empowering?

  o If you catch yourself apologizing automatically, just pause and try again. This isn't about getting it right every time. It's about awareness and practice.

23.

Assemble a Team and Listen to Their Advice

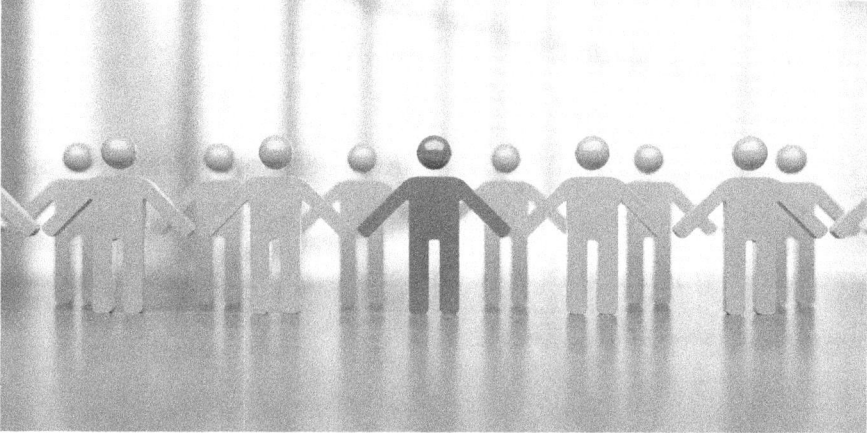

Both parts of this lesson are equally important. Find people who can help AND choose to listen to them.

Thriving after brain injury doesn't happen in a vacuum. It takes support from professionals, family members, friends, and other brain injury survivors. I often say that I'm a group project.

Professionals have helped me heal, taught me strategies, and supported my journey toward accepting both my new self and my new life.

Family and friends have given me shoulders to cry on, caught me when I fell, cheered me on, and stayed by my side.

Other brain injury survivors have offered empathy and validation based on our shared experience. Hearing their stories has made me feel less alone in mine.

At one time or another, every member of my team has told me hard truths when I needed to hear them. They've helped me find resilience, wisdom, and strength. I know I could not have learned to thrive without them.

Assembling a team can feel overwhelming, especially early in the brain injury journey. Finding the right people is a process of trial and error, one that often takes more time than we'd like. For me, it took years to build the team I have now. The process continues as I live and age with brain injury.

When assembling a team, there will be challenges and setbacks along the way.

We may struggle to find the right professionals to help us. It can be difficult, especially in the early years, to know who to trust. Not all professionals are knowledgeable about brain injury and may recommend treatments that don't help or set us back.

We may encounter professionals who don't believe us—who doubt our experience or question the severity of our symptoms. Being disbelieved by those we look to for guidance is devastating.

Some cherished members of our team may relocate, retire, or pass away, leaving painful gaps.

Geography can also be a challenge. The specialists we need may be far from where we live. A local brain injury support group may not exist.

Some friends or family we counted on may disappear from our lives, leaving us emotionally shattered. Hurtful comments from people who don't understand brain injury can cut deep.

Those who do stay by our side often have their own journey to navigate, as they work to understand and adapt to our brain injury. They are grieving too. Patience may be needed—on all sides.

There are also practical obstacles. Insurance might not cover the treatments we need. There may be a gap between what we need and what we can afford.

And even though we are struggling with all the challenges of brain injury, it is likely we will also have to advocate for ourselves to get the help we need.

As I was building my team, many of these challenges took me by surprise. I share them not to discourage you, but to prepare you. Knowing what to expect can make the journey a little easier. Because even with all the difficulties, the benefits of a trusted team are worth it.

Creating a trusted team starts with noticing how people make you feel. Look for those who listen without judgment, believe your experience, and support your journey. Start small; one steady supporter can lead to others. Over time, your team can grow and evolve with you. What matters is finding people who see you, believe in you, and are willing to walk beside you on this path.

But assembling a team is only half the journey. The other half—learning to let their wisdom in—is often just as challenging. It can take years to learn to listen.

In my early years after brain injury, when all I wanted was to return to my old life, I blocked out a lot of good advice from my trusted team. My wall of denial was strong.

I'm grateful for those who kept offering their insight and guidance—gently and in small doses—as I was able to process it during those years. Patience may be needed from our team as we learn to listen.

I'm also grateful for those who were blunt with me when it mattered most, who wouldn't take no for an answer when my safety or well-being was at stake. Persistence may also be needed from our team as we learn to listen.

It wasn't until I moved through denial that I became more open to listening to advice. What I know now is my brain lies to me. I overestimate what I can do and because of that, there are times when my team can see things I can't.

So, when people I trust offer guidance, I weigh it carefully. They care about me and want what's best for me. They're on my team for a reason, and I owe it to them to listen.

Listening to my team has sharpened my own judgment. As I make decisions, I often hear their voices in my head and know what they would say without even asking.

Learning to listen has helped me avoid setbacks, make wiser choices, and manage life with brain injury more effectively.

Building a team takes time and effort. Listening to them is not always easy, but a strong support system can help brain injury survivors thrive.

We gain strength not just in standing, but in standing with others.

Making It Your Own: Applying Silver Learnings

Use this space to reflect on the support systems in your life. The questions and action item below are designed to help you connect your experience to the key ideas from this lesson: building a team, learning to listen, and accepting guidance.

Section 1: Individual Reflection Questions

- Which people have been helpful to me in my brain injury journey?

- What kind of support do I still need?

- When is it hard for me to take advice?

Section 2: Group Discussion Questions

- How have you found people for your support team?

- Has anyone ever told you something that was hard to hear, but helped you grow?

- How do you decide whether to follow someone else's advice?

Section 3: Action Item—Suggestion for a Next Step after Reading Lesson 23

- Celebrate your Team

  o Think of one person who has supported you well.

  o Reflect on what they've given you—healing, patience, honesty, kindness, encouragement.

  o If you can, thank them in person or on the phone. If not, write a few words of gratitude.

24.

Recognize and Celebrate Progress

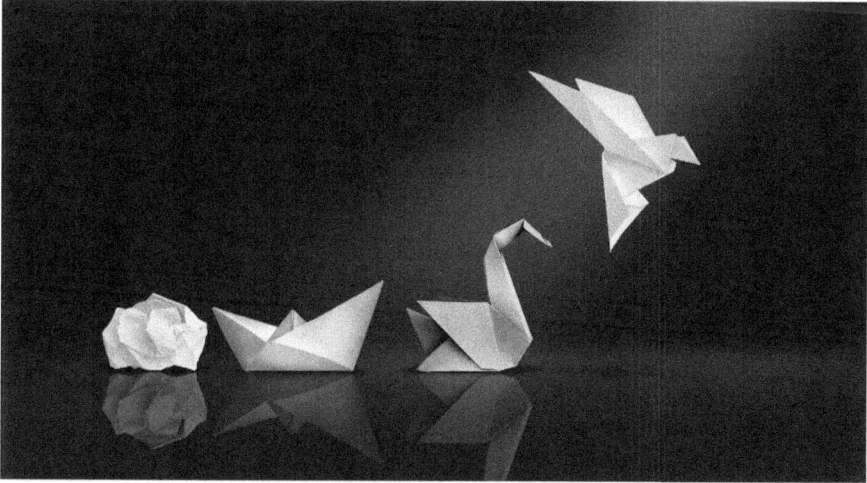

Lightspring/Shutterstock.com

The brain injury journey is full of twists and turns. Sometimes we inch forward and sometimes we slide backward. Sometimes it feels like we're stuck and not moving at all.

During all that twisting, turning, and backsliding, it's easy to get discouraged. It can be hard to see that any progress has been made.

But we do make progress. To quote one of my other *Silver Learning* lessons, *Where you are now is not where you will always be: Change is slow, but possible.*

Each gain we make, no matter how small, changes us. Our progress can be visualized as a series of folds, like the origami shown in the picture on the previous page. Fold by fold, hard-won gain by hard-won gain, we are transformed.

During my early years after brain injury, I felt like I'd been reduced to a crumpled mass, formless and unrecognizable. But even then, transformation was happening. Tiny folds of incremental change were occurring.

Part of thriving is being able to recognize and celebrate those tiny folds.

Noticing and honoring our progress—especially during times of backsliding or increased symptoms—remind us we are still, always, transforming. They can motivate us to keep moving forward, one small fold at a time.

I had a hard time recognizing the progress I made after my brain injury. Because old Carole was my standard, nothing new Carole did was ever good enough. I discounted my gains because they seemed inconsequential compared to who I used to be. Yes, I was much too hard on myself!

Documenting my accomplishments in a portfolio helped me learn to recognize my progress. As I collected mementos of hard-won achievements and gains, I realized there were new Carole accomplishments to be proud of. I was indeed making progress and slowly transforming from crumpled mass to soaring bird.

My portfolio is an archive of my brain injury journey. The back pages highlight achievements that were once challenging and huge wins at the time, such as creating a meal plan and attending a brain injury conference. These are activities I can now do more easily.

Seeing the progression from past to present in my portfolio makes it easy to recognize how far I've come.

My portfolio also reminds me how hard I've worked for the gains I've made. For example, I can now attend classical concerts again. Ticket stubs and notes saved in my portfolio remind me that it took years to achieve that accomplishment.

During times when my own brain injury journey is extra twisty and it's hard to remember how far I've come, my portfolio does that for me. It's now six inches thick of reminders to recognize my progress.

A portfolio is not the only way to document progress. Photos, video recordings, audio recordings, sticky notes, journal writing, social media posts, or blog entries are all ways to capture our experience and provide a record of our journey.

There is power in the act of noticing. When we document changes over time—even if they're small—we can remember that progress <u>is</u> happening, and we <u>are</u> transforming.

Celebrating progress matters too. Every step forward deserves recognition. No gain is too small, no pace too slow. Taking time to celebrate reminds us that progress is unfolding, even when it feels invisible. Celebration can lift our spirits, quiet discouragement, and make space for joy, pride, and gratitude to grow.

I celebrate my progress every year on July 6th, the anniversary of the car accident that caused my brain injury. I know, that seems like an odd day to celebrate. I am not celebrating the fact that I have a brain injury; I am celebrating how far I've come since 1999. One of the ways I celebrate is to look at my portfolio.

Celebrating progress on July 6th is about claiming that day for myself. A lot was taken from me on July 6th, 1999. I did not have a choice in that. But on that day every year, I can choose to celebrate how far I've come, and I can use that celebration to change July 6th from a mournful day to a more positive one.

Brain injury changes everything in a moment. But fold by fold, step by step, we can transform. As we learn to notice and celebrate our progress, we can become stronger, wiser, and more resilient. We can thrive.

Making It Your Own: Applying Silver Learnings

Here is an opportunity to think about the progress you've made since your brain injury. The questions and action item below are designed to help you connect your experience to the key ideas from this lesson: noticing small changes, recognizing transformation over time, and finding meaningful ways to celebrate progress.

Section 1: Individual Reflection Questions

- What is one small gain I've made that I am proud of?

- What could I use to help me notice progress that happens slowly over time?

- What does celebrating progress look like for me?

Section 2: Group Discussion Questions

- How are you different now, compared to the beginning of your brain injury journey?

- How does hearing about each other's progress help you reflect on your own?

- Have you found ways to celebrate how far you've come? What has worked for you?

Section 3: Action Item—Suggestion for a Next Step after Reading Lesson 24

- Mark One Fold: Honor a Small Transformation

  o Choose one small, but meaningful gain you've made since your brain injury.

  o Take one of the following steps to mark it:
    - Take a photo or a screenshot of it
    - Write a note, card, or journal entry about it
    - Tell someone about it
    - Add it to a box, file, or folder

  o The purpose is to notice one small sign, one reminder that progress is happening and you are transforming.

of suffering. Making meaning can transform loss into resilience, empathy, strength, wisdom, and personal growth.

There are many ways to begin. You might share your story in a support group, reflect through journaling or art, help someone in need, spend time in nature, or connect with your spiritual or religious practice.

Purpose is meaning put into action. Often, we find it where our talents, passions, and values meet.

As brain injury survivors, we can discover our talents, passions, and values by getting to know our new selves, focusing on what we can do, and taking risks. Like everything else with brain injury, finding meaning and purpose takes time, it takes patience, and it takes effort.

Purpose may be big, bold, or public like advocating for a cause, writing a book, or speaking at events. But purpose can also live in quiet moments, such as being there for a loved one, creating something for oneself, or taking care of a pet or plant. Finding purpose is a personal journey.

Connecting with a sense of purpose can bring meaning to our days, provide motivation to get up in the morning, bring feelings of fulfillment and belonging, inspire us to set goals, and encourage us to move forward.

There can even be health benefits to having a sense of purpose, including better sleep, lower stress levels, a healthier immune system, and improved cognition.

Over my years of living with brain injury, I have found meaning through helping other survivors. Because I am still a teacher at heart, my actions lean toward the educational. I have found purpose as a brain injury speaker, author, group leader, and mentor. This has become my life's work.

This final lesson about making meaning from suffering is not the end of the story, but the beginning of something new. It is a foundation for the new life we're building, a life where grief can turn into growth and struggle can lead to strength.

We may not have chosen this brain injury path, but we can choose what we make of it. And in that choice, we begin to frame our story and find the light.

Making meaning and connecting to purpose may not erase the darkness that is brain injury, but they can help us shine in spite of it.

Making It Your Own: Applying Silver Learnings

This final reflection section invites you to think about your path forward after brain injury. The questions and action item below are designed to help you connect your experience to the key ideas from this lesson: making intentional choices, finding meaning after brain injury, and taking small steps toward finding purpose.

Section 1: Individual Reflection Questions

- Have I made the choice to find meaning in my life after brain injury?

- What part of my life feels most meaningful right now?

- What do I enjoy that could help me find purpose?

Section 2: Group Discussion Questions

- Does thinking about meaning and purpose change how you think about your brain injury? If so, how?

- What choices can you make that will help you find meaning and purpose?

- Have you developed a sense of purpose since your brain injury?

Section 3: Action Item—Suggestion for a Next Step after Reading Lesson 25

- Begin to *Make Something*

  o Let the words *make something* guide you. What could you create, begin, or offer to others right now? Here are some possibilities:
    ▪ Start a small creative project like a drawing, photo, essay, poem, or handmade card
    ▪ Begin a meaning journal to write or sketch what gives your life value today
    ▪ Put together a music playlist that reflects your healing journey
    ▪ Plant something as a symbol of ongoing growth
    ▪ Create a small visual reminder of your purpose, such as a word/picture collage, decorated stone, or note on your mirror

  o Reflect: *What did this act of making something show me about where I am now and where I want to go?*

CONCLUSION

The Journey Continues...

I write this conclusion as my twenty-fifth year of living with brain injury draws to a close. That silver milestone inspired me to weave the threads of my experience together, first into a speech, and then this book. I hope the reflections, insights, and strategies I've shared have encouraged you to explore your own journey.

Whether you've read one lesson or all twenty-five, you've taken a step toward understanding, accepting, and honoring your experience.

No matter where you are on the brain injury path, there is value in reflecting, in pausing to think about your journey. You don't have to wait for a milestone like twenty-five years. Reflection can be an ongoing practice.

Reflection can bring clarity. Looking back can help you better understand your experience and make informed choices about the road ahead.

Reflection can build self-compassion. Pausing to think about your journey is an opportunity to treat yourself with kindness and respect.

Reflection can support growth. By noticing what has been difficult and what has gone well, you gain insight. That insight can help you move forward with strength and resilience.

Our lives are richly woven tapestries. Reflection invites you to pull on some of your threads, to see what patterns emerge. The threads I've shared in this book are silver, in honor of my twenty-five years. Yours may be any color you choose.

My book ends here, but the journey does not. There is no final chapter to life after brain injury. We can continue to learn about ourselves, deepen our understanding of brain injury, and find ways to move forward in our new lives for the rest of our days.

May your journey continue with strength, meaning, and hope. And may you find your own silver learnings along the way.

ACKNOWLEDGMENTS

The lessons in this book are silver threads, woven together from my twenty-five years of living with brain injury. But threads alone don't make a fabric. A strong backing is also needed for support. This book exists because of all the people who have nurtured, guided, protected, encouraged, and supported me over the years.

Special thanks go to Rorie Lee, Ross Goldberg, and Hilary Zayed, my amazing writing group and wonderful friends. They brought to this book the layered perspectives of brain injury survivors, caregivers, writers, artists, teachers, mentors, and philosophers. Our writing retreat conversations helped clarify my thinking, and their honest, thoughtful critiques pushed my writing to a higher level. I am grateful for their wisdom, encouragement, and belief in this book—and in me.

Thank you to my sister Mary Starr and dear friend Gail Wormwood for giving the book the final once-over before publication, looking for stray typos, correcting formatting issues, and offering valuable feedback.

Brain injury didn't just happen to me; it affected everyone in my circle. I am eternally grateful for the unwavering support of my family and dear friends. They have given me shoulders to cry on, rescued me when I overloaded, provided tough love when needed, acted as sounding boards, helped me create this new life, cheered my successes, travelled with me, attended my speeches, stayed by me, and so much more. I owe much of my resilience to them and know I could not have progressed this far without their assistance. With much love, I thank Donald Starr, Serena Wakelin-Starr, Mary Starr, Kerem Durdag, Kemal Durdag, Sofia Durdag, Lila Durdag, Sylvia Wallingford, Gail Wormwood, Rorie Lee, Ross Goldberg, Hilary Zayed, and Bethany Bryan.

Sadly, my mother Joyce Starr passed away before the publication of *Silver Learnings* or my first book, *To Root & To Rise: Accepting Brain Injury*. In the early years after my brain injury, my mother went with me to many medical appointments. She also sat beside me the day I gave my first five-minute speech about brain injury. I am forever grateful for her never-ending love, gentle wisdom, and fierce devotion to helping me create a new life after brain injury. I know she would be proud of everything I have accomplished.

My mentor Bev Bryant also passed away before the publication of either book. Bev lit a path for me as a brain injury survivor, speaker, and author. Through her words and deeds, she taught me how to be a mentor and a group leader. She believed in my ability to use my experience to make a difference. It is now my privilege to continue Bev's legacy and strive to be a light to other brain injury survivors the way she was a light to me.

The people who best understand the brain injury journey are those who live it every day. Other brain injury survivors have validated my experience, provided empathy, and made me feel less alone. It has been a joy and privilege to work with survivors in Maine and across the country to use our stories to make a difference. I am grateful for all I've learned over the years from the members of the WINGS Brain Injury Support Group and my colleagues in Brain Injury Voices and the Brain Injury Association of America's Brain Injury Advisory Council.

Professionals have taught me strategies to cope with my challenges, encouraged me as I built a new life and helped me continue to heal. Special thanks to those who have traveled this road with me the longest—Denise Toppi, LMT, PTA (Massage Therapy), Dr. Keelyn Wu, DO (Osteopathy), and Lindy Grigel, MHP, PA-C, CCH (Homeopathy). Their knowledge, care, and wisdom have made a profound difference in my life.

I owe a great deal to the many professionals, both past and present, who have influenced my brain injury journey. With deep gratitude, I thank the following people and organizations:

Paul Albert, PT

Dr. Nathan Corbell, PhD, OD

Eliza Dorsey, OT

Dr. Stephen Goldbas, DO

Marjorie Haney, PT

Dr. Heidi Henninger, MD

Dr. Vincent Herzog, DO

Dr. Leigh Ann Higgins, MD

Nancy King, RDH

Dr. James Kirsh, DO

Kathy Kroll, CTRS

Eric Laszlo, NASM, CPT

Kelly Lynch, MA, CCC-A

Susan Marcet, LICSW, ACSW

Dr. William Maxwell, MD

Dr. David Merrill, MD

Diana Page, ACNP

Dr. Colin Robinson, OD

Dr. Megan Selvitelli, MD

Alison van Zandbergen, RN, CBP

James Varmecky, PT

Goodwill NeuroRehab Services

New England Rehabilitation Hospital of Portland

If I have unintentionally left anyone out, please accept both my apologies and my heartfelt thanks.

APPENDIX

Making It Your Own **Page Numbers**

Use this appendix to quickly locate the individual reflection questions, group discussion questions, and action items from each chapter.

About the Author

Carole J. Starr, M.S., is a brain injury survivor, national keynote speaker, author, group leader, and mentor. Before her injury, Carole was building a career as an educator and performing as an amateur violinist and singer.

A car accident in 1999 changed everything. Carole had to give up her profession and her hobbies. In the years that followed, she grieved the loss of her old life and identity. Slowly and with support, she began to rebuild by focusing on what she *could* do. Step by step, she created a new life and a new purpose.

Today, Carole uses her lived experience to educate, advocate, and support others living with brain injury. She is the author of *To Root & To Rise: Accepting Brain Injury* and *Silver Learnings: Practical Wisdom for Living with Brain Injury*. Carole presents at brain injury conferences across the country, facilitates a brain injury support group, and has held leadership roles in state and national brain injury groups.

Through her writing, speaking, and leadership, Carole has found a new way to be a teacher. She is committed to making a difference and helping others find strength, meaning, and hope after brain injury.

Visit StarrSpeakerAuthor.com to contact Carole, read excerpts from her books, and watch videos of her speeches.

www.ingramcontent.com/pod-product-compliance
Lightning Source LLC
LaVergne TN
LVHW051503080426
835509LV00017B/1903